SACRAMENTO PUBLIC LIBRARY
828 "I" Street
Sacramento, CA 95814
01/14

FOREVER BEAUTIFUL

The Age-Defying Detox Plan

NATALIA ROSE

Guilford, Connecticut
An imprint of Globe Pequot Press

To buy books in quantity for corporate use
or incentives, call **(800) 962-0973**
or e-mail **premiums@GlobePequot.com**.

skirt!® is an attitude . . . spirited, independent, outspoken, serious, playful and irreverent, sometimes controversial, always passionate.

Copyright © 2014 by Natalia Rose

ALL RIGHTS RESERVED. No part of this book may be reproduced or transmitted in any form by any means, electronic or mechanical, including photocopying and recording, or by any information storage and retrieval system, except as may be expressly permitted in writing from the publisher. Requests for permission should be addressed to Globe Pequot Press, Attn: Rights and Permissions Department, P.O. Box 480, Guilford, CT 06437.

skirt!® is an imprint of Globe Pequot Press
skirt! ® is a registered trademark of Morris Publishing Group, LLC, and is used with express permission.

Illustrations by Nina Duran
Text design: Sheryl P. Kober
Layout: Sue Murray
Project editor: Ellen Urban

Library of Congress Cataloging-in-Publication Data is available on file.

ISBN 978-0-7627-8085-3

Printed in the United States of America

10 9 8 7 6 5 4 3 2 1

This book is written as a source of information only. The health and diet information contained in this book is based solely on the personal and professional experiences of the author and is not intended as a medical manual. The information should not be used for diagnosis or treatment, or as a substitute for professional medical care.

For my mother, Rita Barrett,
who is forever beautiful

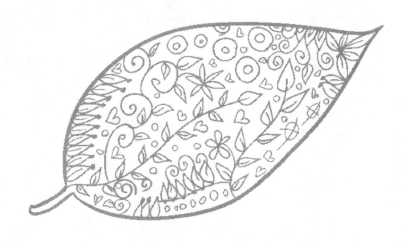

CONTENTS

Contents

Contents

FOREWORD

You are about to experience the power of nutritional greatness and the glory of detoxification. You are about to amplify the innate intelligence of your body.

Dr. Sara Gottfried here. I'm a Harvard-educated physician, an MIT bioengineer, and the author of the best-selling book *The Hormone Cure: Reclaim Balance, Sleep, Sex Drive and Vitality Naturally with the Gottfried Protocol.* Not least of all, I'm a yoga instructor, mom, wife, and enthusiastic champion of health, happiness, and hormonal harmony.

I've spent the last two decades of my life trying to change the way we approach medicine. Instead of going straight from symptoms to diagnosis to prescription, I take a more integrated approach that focuses on preventative measures, finding the root cause of the issue, and using as little artificial medication as possible.

On this point, Natalia Rose and I are in strong alignment: While Western medication certainly has its place, too many people are searching for the magic pharmaceutical that will solve all their problems. What Natalia and I have each discovered separately is that the silver bullet exists—it's just not found at the bottom of a prescription pill bottle. Instead, most of us just need to make small changes to the way we live our lives, eradicating the toxic elements and replacing them with rejuvenating ones.

I first became aware of Natalia Rose's work when I started to research longevity, aging, and how to naturally fight back against the stressors of modern living. When you run a business focused on balancing the hormones of middle-aged women, can you see that this topic might come up a lot? What I love about Natalia's message is that it is based both on proven strategies and a holistic view of health and the human body—one that I think many of us have lost in the frantic rush of modern life. And if you know anything about me, know this: I am a stickler for the science. I pull from ancient proven practices (meditation, Ayurveda, acupuncture) as well as the most cutting-edge science we have on botanical supplements and bioidentical hormones.

In *Forever Beautiful,* readers get strategies and tips for living in a way that is more fulfilling and, let's face it, a far more revitalizing beauty routine than loading our faces with toxic chemicals. Natalia makes the important point that our current lifestyle is one that actually accelerates aging—the very thing most of us, especially women, are trying to prevent at all costs! Natalia tackles two main problems in her book:

1. That the modern stereotype of "youthful beauty" is artificial, manu-factured, and causing more harm than good. Aging gracefully is slowly disappearing from today's media-driven world.

2. That our modern lifestyle itself is *causing* accelerated aging—sagging skin, abdominal fat, and bodies sapped of energy and purpose. In a cruel irony, the toxins found in the products we use to prevent the effects of aging are actually contributing to the problem.

Forever Beautiful presents the importance of detoxing, from our cells to our soul, and I agree with this approach wholeheartedly. Because most of our minds, bodies, and environments are laden with toxic elements—from body image to food to furniture—Natalia's advice on how to clean out clogged systems is an important first step. We all get off track sometimes (even the most dedicated yogis and whole-foodists), so I personally detox quarterly. A hormone-balancing detox is also one of the most popular programs I offer my own tribe; I get overwhelmingly positive feedback from women who are amazed at their renewed energy, vigor, and easy weight loss. It is the perfect way to reset hormones and return to a pattern of more-balanced lifestyle choices. Natalia's advice on how to start, what to do, and how to hold on to the rhythm will get many people taking their first important steps toward a healthier body and a more joyful sense of self.

I agree with Dr. Mark Hyman that what's on the end of your fork is more powerful than anything you'll find in a pill bottle. Years of research and study have shown me that diet can be the single greatest determinant of over-all health. Nutrients, fiber, minerals, and vitamins that are consumed daily will have a greater effect and a larger impact on your weight, hormones, and appearance than any prescription or medical procedure. Natalia has written four other books focused on the healing power of food, and the large section of this book devoted to eating for longevity makes me do the happy dance.

Stretching the spine! Eating alkalizing foods! Practicing forgiveness! This is my jam, and Natalia knows just how powerful these practices are. She's been a leader in the natural beauty community for years, and has worked with everyone from celebrities to soccer moms to help create beauty routines and simple daily habits that fight back against environmental toxins, as well as polluted mind-sets. This lady knows the power of the mind/body connection, which is why *Forever Beautiful* goes further than most detox manuals. This isn't just about how to lose weight fast, or how to flush toxins out of your system; this is an in-depth manual for creating a lifestyle that is in harmony with nature, your own personal needs, and the natural aging process.

There are probably some who think that cellular cleansing and electromagnetic energy are a little on the mystical side, but to those skeptics I say, "Give it a try." I'm a Harvard MD who has seen firsthand the difference that a kale smoothie and regular grounding has made in not just my life, but the lives of thousands of patients. I blend the modern and the traditional in the health strategies that I prescribe my patients, and it's exciting to me that women like Natalia are doing the same. The time and heavy research that goes into vetting and testing these techniques is no small feat; you can consider this book a treasure trove of advice on how to achieve timeless beauty.

There's no denying that our modern lifestyle is a problematic one, so when someone like Natalia Rose gives you a book packed with advice and ideas on how to navigate the murky waters of detoxification, aging, and health, you read it.

—*Sara Gottfried, MD, Berkeley, CA*

NOTE TO READER

Legend has it that Thoth, the ancient Atlantean, would lay himself under the fabled Flower of Life for ten out of every thousand years to regenerate his body in order to remain eternally young. Alexander the Great, Ponce de León, and countless other explorers have searched the world over with the hope of finding the Fountain of Youth. Some believe that there exist Taoist Masters in the Himalayas and Shaolin monks who possess these secrets of immortality; some are rumored to have lived for centuries in luminous, youthful bodies.

Are there germs of truth in these legendary accounts? Could it be that we are simply unaware of how to utilize the natural laws of life to restore our bodies and free ourselves from the clutches of physical degradation? Rather than maintaining the status quo, could we be living extraordinary lives in bodies that can be fully vitalized and resplendent for far longer than dictated by our culture? I have researched this subject with the same laser focus I have brought to cellular cleansing, and I say the answer is a resounding yes!

I believe this book holds the crux of this lost knowledge and the principles by which we can revitalize ourselves in today's world. It is my pleasure to share this wisdom with you. May you benefit immensely!

—*Natalia Rose*

INTRODUCTION

Are you feeling prematurely old and tired?

Are you often, or always, disappointed by what you see in the mirror?

Do you fear that your best days are already behind you?

Are you fighting tooth and claw to maintain a youthful appearance?

Do you see time and nature as your enemies?

Does contemplating your age fill you with a sense of dread and futility?

If you've answered yes to any or all of these questions, you're among millions who have fallen prey to a world of misguided notions about youth, beauty, health, and aging. Believe me, I understand. Aging is not for the faint of heart, especially in a world that seems to prize youth and flawless Photoshopped beauty above all other virtues. When you live in an image-conscious, youth-obsessed society, it is painful to look in the mirror and see your face falling. For all the scientific research and technological advances of our modern age, you would think by now we would have found the secret to eternal youth. But no; instead, we are using these so-called tools of progress to dig ourselves ever deeper into ignorance, debt, and premature decay.

I live in the middle of New York City on the Upper East Side of Manhattan, fabled for its impeccably polished society women. Many of these women have come to me over the years seeking help to "keep up appearances" as they get older. The pressure to preserve their beauty and youthfulness is very real for them, often for professional as well as social reasons, and it can fully consume their thoughts. But this is not only true for women in New York, Los Angeles, London, Paris, and other pockets of posh society around the world. The fact is, women and men everywhere, at every socioeconomic level, are more image-conscious than ever. Manhattan socialites and Hollywood mavens seem to lead the pack of fierce anti-aging practitioners, but fighting the aging process is as ubiquitous in our culture as trying to lose weight.

Unfortunately, the temptation to visit the plastic surgeon for the latest lifting, tightening, nipping, tucking, and plumping procedures usually wins out, because very few people today have the wisdom and vision to work *with* nature rather than *against* it. The promise of these "enhancements" just seems too convenient to pass up for those with the means to pay for them. People are seeking that particular look, the one manufactured for them by market forces and reinforced by their peers. And once they set out to acquire it, they find there's no endgame, because as time marches on, their bodies just keep bulging and sagging and wrinkling as new cosmetic drugs and treatments hit the market. These insatiable youth-seekers keep upping the ante, handing their bodies over, piece by piece, to the anti-aging industry.

Do you count yourself among this social set, spending thousands of dollars a year on cosmetic drugs and procedures as a matter of course? Or are you of more modest means, but still spend a significant portion of your monthly paycheck on aggressively marketed over-the-counter products? In either case, it's time to ask yourself: *What's the real price of all this, beyond just a heck of a lot of money?* Because the fact is, while some mainstream anti-aging methods may help to hide certain signs of aging temporarily, almost all of them concurrently accelerate the deterioration of cells and tissues, as well as initiate a vicious cycle that is likely to ensnare a person for life.

In this culture, we perceive ourselves and the aging process through a paradigm of disconnect. Even the term we use, *anti-aging,* betrays a deeply negative, combative approach to our bodies. Meanwhile, we place far too much stock in numbers. We think that what ages us is the number of times we travel around the sun. But what really ages us is how we travel around the sun—more specifically, how much waste and obstruction we accumulate along the way, and how much we either cooperate with the universal laws of life or oppose them.

At the heart of our youth-obsessed culture is an ignorance that has grown out of all proportion with reality; we've forgotten where we come from, how we are made, what we are made of, and how to care for ourselves properly. Sure, we know that humans develop from the union of a sperm and an egg and are incubated for about forty weeks in a woman's uterus before birth, and we know enough technicalities about the physical body to fill volumes of medical textbooks. But where have these catalogs of cold, hard, scientific facts led us? Where is the wisdom and understanding?

In my lifetime, I've known very few people who have consciously chosen a life-generating path in response to aging. Everyone else I've encountered has followed a path of fear—fear of growing old, fear of social rejection, fear of demotion, fear of failure, fear of losing love, fear of surrendering to love and being found out, fear of the truth, fear of laying bare one's authentic self. Everywhere I turn, I see fearful adults who are fighting desperately to turn back the clock and are thereby accelerating the aging process instead. Youthfulness is the flowering of a life-generating path, impossible even for the chronologically young who follow a life-deteriorating route of unnatural consumption.

There is a big difference between the natural aging process, which is inevitable for all life forms, and the modern deterioration that is ravaging our bodies and spirits at warp speeds and sending us into panic mode. If you're only interested in looking camera-ready for the duration of a three-hour event, with a ton of makeup and the trick of soft lighting, then you've come to the wrong place. On the other hand, if you want to learn how to tap into the powerful fountain of youth lying dormant within you, to look and feel positively radiant day in and day out, then you've stumbled upon some unbelievable good luck.

As nature's creatures, we all carry within us a fountain of youth—an immeasurable source of vitality that, if honored, will serve us well throughout a long and fruitful life. We simply need to access it in order to nurture our bodies and souls as we would a garden—gently and holistically, with an abundance of rich soil, fresh air, fresh water, and sunlight. For as long as we are alive, we can choose a life-generating path in order to age not only gracefully, but gorgeously!

The fact is, you cannot hold your radiance when cut off from the source of life any more than a fruit can grow once cut from the vine. If you are like most people today, young or old, you are prematurely plucking yourself from the vine and accelerating decay. I spent the first twenty-plus years of my life doing the same, until I finally woke up to the madness. Ever since, I've devoted myself to a life of healing and regeneration. I've gathered insights into these subjects from a broad spectrum of teachers, books, and what I call "spiritual downloads." I've also gathered many empirical truths from years of experience as a professional nutritionist, dietician, detox specialist, and healing catalyst. Measuring these insights and observations against one another has been my scientific method, and this method has led me to a far stronger paradigm for living than I've found anywhere else.

That is why I've written this book—to help stop the cycles of fear, waste, decay, self-hatred, and suffering associated with aging. Here is what you will find in the following pages:

- In Part I, we will delve right into the core natural law that is absolutely fundamental to timeless beauty, or what I often refer to as youth regeneration. This natural law, and all the wisdom that springs from it, will give you a whole new outlook on aging.

- Then, in Part II, I introduce the five main principles of timeless beauty—all firmly rooted in the core natural law—along with the most effective and practical ways to apply them to your lifestyle. Together, these principles and their applications make up the powerful age-defying detox method for revitalizing your whole life.

- In Part III, I share with you a series of my favorite facial exercises, a gentle but effective way to tone the contours of the face for a more youthful appearance.

- Then, in Part IV, I provide a three-week plan for those of you who seek a guided initiation to practicing the age-defying detox method. This is the same protocol I recommend for my age-conscious clients. I guarantee that with consistent application, your whole state of being—physical, emotional, mental, and spiritual—will be renewed!

- In Part V, I answer many questions about the phenomena of modern aging, covering diseases, sexuality, bone integrity, mental decline, hormone replacement therapy, and so much more.

- In Part VI, I interview seven of today's leading health practitioners and pioneering minds on solutions to modern aging.

- You will find the recipe section in Part VII, where I unveil new recipes to help make every meal cleansing, rejuvenating, and joyful.

- Finally, don't miss the Forever Beautiful Shopping Guide at the end of the book!

So come with me. Get off the depressing hamster wheel of commercial anti-aging trends and discover the power of your own indwelling fountain of youth!

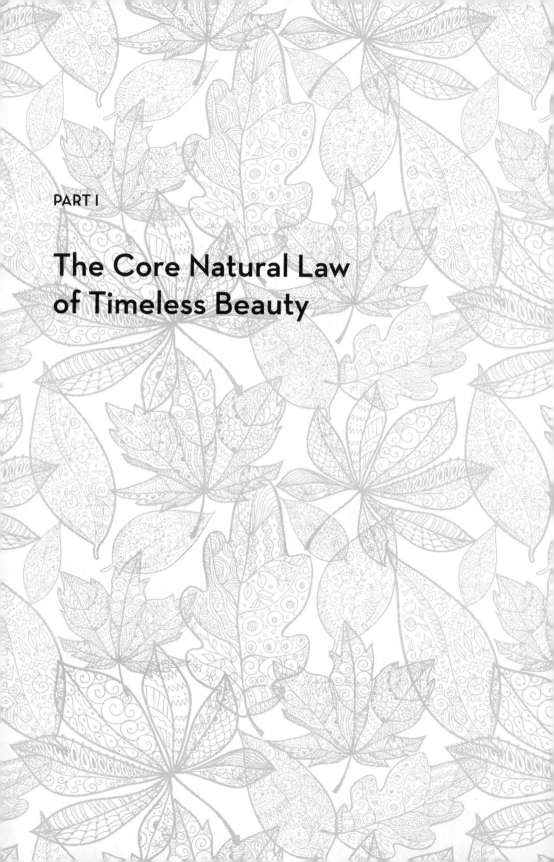

PART I

The Core Natural Law of Timeless Beauty

Every time you strive to improve on Nature by going against it, you will damage yourself, for Nature is your very being." Consider this quote by one of our great spiritual thinkers, Anthony de Mello, and then consider that virtually everything we do, buy, and consume in our mainstream culture opposes or attempts to control nature. Then notice that almost all of it is presented as an improvement upon nature. What we keep forgetting, at every turn, is that any life lived out of sync with nature is doomed.

Now, let's take this concept and retool it to speak more positively and directly to rejuvenation: *To experience the grace and vitality of youth, we must flow with nature, not against it.*

I urge you to make this your mantra. If you engage this core natural law, if you commit to truly understanding and internalizing it, the power of expanded consciousness and focused intent will transform every aspect of your life. Every single principle and application you will learn in this book supports this law.

The typical symptoms of aging—such as stiffness, weight gain, energy loss, depression, aches and pains, to name just a few—are not as irreparable as most people think. If they were, then nature wouldn't be very powerful. We can be thankful that Mother Nature is as immeasurably powerful as she is, and that we all carry her power within us, even if it's long been suppressed or dormant. If there remains a glimmer of life force in the body, there's a way to revive it, to give it all the oxygen it needs to bring it back to roaring life. We can regenerate our cells, tissues, organs, and overall appearance, but first, we must dissolve our self-imposed limitations.

Again, this core natural law—*To experience the grace and vitality of youth, we must flow with nature, not against it*—will prove to be our philosopher's stone, the alchemical fulcrum that transforms our deterioration into regeneration, our lead into gold! Once we fully grasp this natural law, it will become clear why the way we typically live and combat aging in the modern world leads to unsightly deterioration and suffering. Or, in other words, why there is no quicker path to physical deterioration than denatured living.

We oppose nature with almost everything we do, from the moment we wake to the moment we fall asleep. In our busy modern lives, we've forgotten how to breathe, much less how to feed and care for ourselves effectively.

Here is just a sampling of some behaviors common to our cultural paradigm that age us prematurely:

We stuff our intestines with processed and acidic foods laden with additives and preservatives.

We take pharmaceutical drugs to suppress symptoms of common illnesses.

We clog our pores with chemical products.

We interrupt our circadian rhythms with too much stress and too little sleep.

We seal ourselves up in airless houses and blast our air conditioners.

We work for a person, institution, or company we don't respect.

We deny our innermost feelings and harbor resentments to keep certain relationships alive.

We overeat, drink, or shop compulsively when we feel sad, stressed, or empty.

Is it any wonder, then, that we, as a modern people, are insulting our own natures and aging so gracelessly? How do we stop living like this? We have to understand that nature is not "over there" while we are "over here." Nature is in the very fabric of our beings, just as each of us is an integral part of the vast fabric of life. We are composed of many interconnected physical systems (skeletal, muscular, nervous, circulatory, respiratory, digestive, and excretory) made up of living cells and energetic patterns designed to operate in a constant flow of communication. But so many of our cultural conditionings create blockages, cutting off this flow of communication and devitalizing our systems.

It's not too late to become wise to nature's patterns and laws. In the most natural habitats still left on Earth we find life in all its ingenious glory, exhibiting strength, sensitivity, flexibility, intuition, movement, and beauty.

Notice that most children also have these qualities: strong wills and strong cellular integrity, but sensitive natures, flexible limbs, and intuitive minds; an ease and joy in their movements; effortless, unself-conscious beauty. My son likes to show me how he can jump hard but land softly. We can learn so much from children who have not yet been completely denatured!

Mental Exercise

To experience the grace and vitality of youth, we must flow with nature, not against it. *Find a quiet moment to sit with this core natural law for a moment. Repeat it to yourself several times slowly. As simple as this concept may seem, really let it sink into your consciousness. Then look at your world in light of it. Look at your immediate surroundings. Look at yourself. Look at your daily routines—at your work, your home, your social environment. Think about your last ten purchases. Think about the last ten things you consumed. Did they promote the flow of nature or oppose it? Is there a natural flow to your life, or do you experience much struggle and interference? Do you carry a lot of tension?* To experience the grace and vitality of youth, we must flow with nature, not against it. *Come back to this concept as often as you need to. Let it be the harbinger of your regeneration!*

We adults, on the other hand, have been "civilized" away from these innate qualities and mainstreamed into consumer culture. Every directive of this culture programs us to work, spend, and consume our way to wealth, beauty, and happiness. Of course, we'll never quite get there, because modern notions of wealth, beauty, and happiness are marketed illusions designed to keep us working, spending, consuming, acquiring, and accumulating our lives away. So most of us move through life like automatons, mindlessly colluding with life-deteriorating norms, letting them steadily chip away at our most prized possession—our vitality, or our life force. We yearn with all our hearts for youth and beauty, prosperity and strength, clarity and joy—yet we go about it all wrong, breaking our backs and spirits in the process. And so we yearn for them all the more, breaking ourselves down further in this endlessly misguided pursuit.

There is nothing natural about aging in the modern world. It's misleading to call it aging—more accurately, what we're seeing is abnormal deterioration, decay, degeneration, mutation. Most tragic of all, we begin this process of decay the moment we are born. From day one, we inherit these unnatural paradigms for living and are forced to sacrifice our beauty and youthfulness—indeed, our whole biochemistry—to the silent and not-so-silent ravages of our world.

If we were living in harmony with natural law, our bodies would still change and show signs of aging, but they would not be the unsightly aberrations that we see today. To avoid confusion, let's call it "modern deterioration." It's an accelerated, mutated version of aging, and it's the result of toxic living. Since nature is our very being, when we oppose nature, we slowly but surely destroy ourselves. Eventually, it all manifests in unseemly ways. Here are some of the most common symptoms:

- Dramatic thinning, sagging, wrinkling, and creasing of skin in the face, neck, and décolletage

- Weight gain, especially in the abdomen

- Under-eye puffiness and discoloration

- Constipation and foul bowel activity

- Chronic fatigue and interrupted sleep

- Bad breath and body odor

- Dwindling sex drive

It is never too late or too early to wake up and step into the light. However many times you've traveled around the sun, you can always begin to regenerate and rejuvenate. You can decide today to stop trading in your power for all the worthless things the modern world says you need, and reconnect with nature's wellspring of vitality. Instead of running around trying to measure up to other people's standards of youth and beauty like a puppet on strings, you can reclaim your autonomy. But it will require a deep perceptual shift.

YOUTH V. AGE

What is it about youth that captures our hearts and imaginations? Youth is fundamentally a state of flowing and blossoming. It is dewy and rosy and delicate and fragrant. Youth is hope, promise, potential. It is beauty, flexibility, irrepressible joy, and inspiration. Pure positive energy. The age-defying detox method revitalizes and reinforces these qualities.

What is the opposite of youth? Obstruction and calcification, of both mind and body. There is nothing youthful about a face-lift. However, much is youthful about a glowing face with gentle laugh lines and a healthful upward lift of expression. A face that has undergone cosmetic surgery often appears frozen, with an unnatural tightness and sheen, whereas a naturally maturing face can be radiant, alive, full of promise.

You can begin right now to tap into your innate youthfulness, those surges of vitality that yearn to flow freely. Remember, life is change, and your cells are constantly changing however you treat them, reflecting the way you live. It's up to you whether they calcify and expire before their time, or if they continually regenerate and rejuvenate. You are a dynamic network of self-reflecting cells and energies—physical and energetic systems that determine your visage, your organs, your blood chemistry. You are only as old as the condition of the cells that comprise your body and the trajectories of thought that guide your life choices. Youth is as much a state of mind as of body.

AGING = ACCUMULATION

When the accumulation of years starts to show, desperation hits. For some, the mere anticipation of the first signs of aging drives them to cosmetic counters and doctors' offices. These anxious types, many of whom are only in their twenties and thirties, are often referred to by cosmetic surgeons and dermatologists as "line chasers." They rush to have every line and flaw filled, lasered, chemically peeled, or otherwise medically treated. It can become an addiction, like compulsive shopping or compulsive exercising. Some people get such a high from manipulating their looks that they keep wanting more and more of that fix. The problem is, you cannot fight nature and win.

If you are addicted to mainstream anti-aging methods, the biggest challenge will be shifting your perspective and adopting an alternative approach. But once you start to see the folly of "line chasing"—how it serves the cosmetic industry far better than it will ever serve you—you will begin to shed the oppressive desperation that has been holding you hostage to it.

While simple aging is a natural event, modern aging reflects decades of toxic accumulation. It's the body groaning under the weight and stress and chemicals that have been imposed upon it. But remember, nature is always at work, either generating life or decomposing it. What we call aging today is accelerated internal and external decomposition due to extreme toxicity—living in opposition to natural law. The falling face, dull complexion, sagging skin, and bulging midsection—these are not natural to a body that has merely circled the sun forty, fifty, or sixty or more times. It is the result of toxic accumulation and the destruction of cellular integrity.

Your body does not choose to ingest the substances that clog its passageways, enflame its organs, and leach its bones. You, the captain of this vessel, make these choices day in and day out. If you are like most people today, you are literally suffocating your own life force, obstructing its natural flow, and thus triggering decay throughout your body. Modern aging is a dire state of decay. The extreme toxicity filling the bloodstream, colon, and organs causes mutations in the body—internally and externally. You can see it with your eyes. That's why treating only surface appearances is a waste of time and money, and often dangerous. Premature aging in the modern world commonly occurs for the following reasons:

- A daily diet of processed foods, meats, and other low-vibration substances

- Overuse of prescription and over-the-counter drugs

- Recreational alcohol and drug abuse

- Radiation from our technocratic world

- Sedentary lifestyles

- High stress levels and lack of sleep

- Invasive medical procedures

The sad fact is, as citizens of the modern world, most of us were born at a disadvantage. Our parents and our parents' parents have passed down to us a genetic and cultural blueprint for toxic living, and in turn, unless we make some dramatic changes, we will pass along those weakened torches to our offspring. This is why you'll often see kids and teens who already have bags and dark circles under their eyes, along with symptoms and diseases formerly common only to adults—such as migraines, arthritis, osteoporosis, and diabetes. Such symptoms indicate internal sluggishness and clogged pathways. Hence, the principles and practices of timeless beauty are not just for the over-forty set. Even the youngest among us are aging prematurely, due to the way we typically live today. It's never too early to introduce ourselves and our children to the natural laws.

FEAR OF AGING

There is no greater hindrance to increased perception than fear. We've all been guilty of closing our eyes to the realities we fear—or, perhaps worse, letting fear direct our choices. There's a great old saying: What you fear most will come upon you. The more you energize a thought, the more you pull it out from the etheric world into the physical world. Nothing will age you quite like the fear of aging. What we resist persists. What we resist we feed with our energy. So if we are focused on fighting aging, we are in effect feeding and accelerating the aging process. If, instead, we focus on generating vitality, on promoting the flow of youth, we will breathe new life into our old selves.

Here's a challenge for you: Try to stop even *thinking* about aging. Stop following gossip magazines and other media outlets that track celebs and reality stars—they promote some of the most insidious, self-defeating messages in your subconscious. They wire you for insecurity, self-judgment, fear, unhealthy comparison, and endless mental chatter that turns your brain to a soup of negativity and dissonance. This translates directly to your life choices, wreaking energy-draining havoc on your cells, tissues, and organs. Yes, the cells and energetic fields of the body can be weakened and disfigured by energy-draining perspectives.

When you overcome your fear, instead of just feeling crushing disappointment at your physical deterioration, you can open your eyes to the cause of that deterioration and let that knowledge spring you into positive action.

> ### Fear Exercise
> Find a quiet, private moment to ask yourself some tough questions.
> Being as honest with yourself as you can, ask yourself the following:
>
> Do I live in a cage of fear?
> Am I terrified of aging?
> What might I lose if my face falls slack or gets more wrinkles?
> What do I think other people see when they look at me?
> What judgments do I think they are making?
> Do I agree with those judgments?
> What are beauty and youthfulness worth to me?
> Who am I trying to please?
> What would I be willing to sacrifice to look younger?
> What wouldn't I be willing to sacrifice?

Now keep in mind that these fears and concerns that disturb your peace of mind reflect only today's truths. If you open yourself up to profound perceptual change, they needn't be tomorrow's! But you must begin with honesty. I recently discussed the topic of youth regeneration on one of our Detox The World radio broadcasts with a consciousness healer, my dear friend Macha Einbender. She shared an exercise that has helped to free her from her own cage of fear. She was kind enough to share it with us here.

Macha's Truth Exercise

Take a pen and notepad and write down everything about yourself that you don't usually like to admit but that you know is true. Your truths may be big or small, rational or irrational, but be really, really honest with yourself. For example, when I did this exercise, I wrote things down such as "I still see myself as a chubby thirteen-year-old" and "I sometimes fear that everyone else is smarter than me." If it helps, start small, and then gradually open up to deeper and deeper truths. Some of them will be painful, but I found this exercise to be ultimately very liberating. Sometimes you have to "out" your ego. Once you bring those things you fear about yourself into the light of day, they become less scary. And from there you can begin to exercise self-compassion and self-empowerment.

So much of what we fear about aging is what we fear about ourselves. This is because we've come to internalize the world we live in, and by the same token, to project our inner demons on the world. A world that devalues nature is, in a word, *destructive*. In this light, why wouldn't we be afraid of it, and afraid of ourselves? Aging, by the modern definition of it, is terrifying indeed. If we have fallen into the trap of fear, it is forgivable. But once we become aware of it, it's our responsibility to do everything it takes to pull ourselves up and out of the darkness, and begin to value ourselves for what we are: living, breathing, dynamic creatures of immeasurable regenerative power.

If you were to ask me what I value most in life, I might easily say my three delectable children and my loving husband. But I would have to explain that this value is neither fixed nor finite. We can only ever value human life as far as the limits of our perception. I'm always seeking to expand my perception from the core natural law. I can only see, feel, conduct, and give as much of myself as far as my perceptual powers allow me to. So, in a sense, what I value most of all is my perception, or my consciousness, for it makes everything else in my life possible.

If you're feeling old and tired and drab, as if your whole life could use a face-lift, resolve to join forces with nature. Resolve to stop fighting and start flowing with that powerful current. This is no time to "double down" against nature, with all manner of expensive chemical products and invasive procedures. It's time to listen to that voice deep within you that knows there's a far better and gentler way to travel around the sun.

SELF-EMPOWERMENT

This is your life, your body, and these are your days. You have to wake up to yourself every day and live your life. You have to inhabit your skin and move through the demands of your world. No one else is going to look after you. Corporations, governments, institutions of medicine and science—they all have their own agendas. Choose self-empowerment, not "hope in a bottle" or the promises of a glossy medical brochure.

You may need to experience many disappointments before you finally realize that injections, laser treatments, surgeries, and expensive chemical creams will never help you to radiate vitality. But sooner or later, if you want real results—ones that can stand up to the tests of time and honest self-assessment—you'll have to be proactive. In this day and age, to flow with the natural order requires consciously stepping out from the misguided herd.

Few industries are growing as rapidly as those of cosmetics and cosmetic medicine. The beauty industry in the United States alone pulls in tens of billions of dollars a year, with the biggest companies routinely reporting rising quarterly profits. Yet I cannot emphasize to you strongly enough that the cosmetic sciences are working diligently to defy and manipulate nature—not to work in harmony with it. Don't be fooled by all the marketing that would have you believe otherwise. It should be illegal to market products and treatments that deteriorate the integrity of the cells, but it's not. The cosmetics industry should be better regulated, but it's not. Why? Because too much money is to be made from them.

For example, teeth whiteners weaken the teeth; synthetic perfumes, lotions, and countless other popular beauty products fill the bloodstream with poisons and infiltrate the organs, contributing to toxic accumulation and sagging skin; topical ointments seep toxins directly into the same cells that they're supposed to be helping, obstructing their absorption of oxygen and the ability to conduct life force. We are mutating our cells and clogging our pathways with every carefully applied product!

Reconnecting with our life force is critical to rejuvenation and wellness of any kind. We cannot forget this. Speaking purely physically, cells cannot be pert and spherical and active if they are not properly fed and oxygenated. Under typical modern conditions, our cells are suffocating and aging long before their time. We are literally cutting them off from vital energy sources. Every plant that flourishes receives its life force through a strong root system. The moment it is cut off from that source, it begins to die. We, too, need constant sources of clean air, water, sunshine, and nutrients to thrive, and we need clear passageways to receive them. These sources are not as easy to tap as they once were, given the increased pollution and contamination of our world, but they are worth our every effort to clean and reconnect with them.

What's more, radiation from our technocratic world is constantly sending dissonant energy waves throughout our bodies, warping our cells and tissues at a subatomic level. We are so much a part of this dissonant soup that it's easy to forget it, but like tuning forks our cells are always absorbing the vibratory notes of our environment. If you are waiting for research to confirm this, you are only delaying bad news, and what you don't know will still affect you. Dissonance is antithetical to life. Track down all the causes of dissonance to every level of your being. Rejuvenation is all about restoring yourself to a state of harmony. It's not just about being beautiful, but living beautifully.

Before moving ahead to the principles and practices of timeless beauty, I would just like to say that they have enhanced my life experience so dramatically for the better that I'll let nothing stand in the way of integrating them into my daily life. They are principles I aim to embody moment to moment. When I succeed at this, the moments of my life string together beautifully with an unparalleled grace; when I don't, disconnect and discordance and chaos ensue.

These principles keep me in such a state of internal harmony and self-empowerment that I can stand firm in the face of misguided social pressures. As a very busy wife and working mother of three kids, I could easily plead stress and exhaustion and let myself unravel without anyone else batting an eye. I could sign up for all kinds of anti-aging treatments and purchase all kinds of expensive products, as my peers do. Making such excuses and choices are considered normal in our world. But I know that nothing compares to feeling alive and youthful in my own skin, and that artificial fixes lead only to accelerated deterioration.

More often than not, I feel wonderful—and, hey, I think I look wonderful too. Not because I fit the world's mold, but because I fit nature's mold. I honor my body and my body honors me back with nature's blessings. I'm not searching outside myself for the fountain of youth; it flows within me. Observing the core natural law of timeless beauty simplifies and harmonizes my life choices, keeping me clear and strong:

To experience the grace and vitality of youth, we must flow with nature, not against it.

Got it?

Good.

Now that you've internalized this core natural law, let's move on to the five principles of timeless beauty and their practical applications.

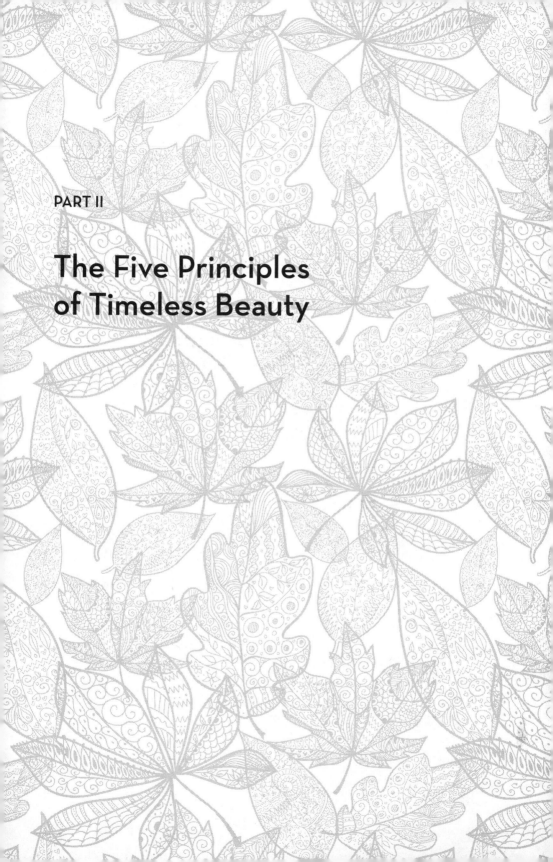

PART II

The Five Principles
of Timeless Beauty

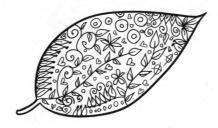

As you consider these principles, note that each one redeems all levels of your being—physical, spiritual, mental, and emotional—to perfect attunement. Each principle is distinct and comes with its own set of practices while, at the same time, reflecting the wisdom of all the others. I encourage you to begin by applying the principles that appeal most to you, and gradually include the others over time, keeping in mind that they all play a key role in the age-defying detox method. This method works best when each and every facet is applied in harmony, but do not force yourself to take on more than you can gracefully apply at once.

I'm going to present one principle at a time, and then recommend practical applications to support them. Gradually, these principles will become an integral part of your knowledge base and not something you have to think about consciously all the time. They'll become a way to perceive and understand rejuvenation, and thus help guide you toward wise, intuitive choices. Just remember, hold on lightly to today's truth, for your perceptions should always be expanding and evolving with experience. Timeless beauty requires not only seeing clearly, but also being prepared to respond to what you see, to make agile adjustments.

Again, just start with what comes most naturally to you, as minimal as that might seem, knowing that when the time is right, the other principles will follow. Don't rush, but do continue to move forward. This is how you'll gain momentum and catch the next wave of vitality—and the next, and the next, and the next!

1. THE PRINCIPLE OF CLARITY

The first step to regeneration, regaining clarity, sounds quite simple, but is actually quite tricky for most people nowadays. You might think your eyes are already open to what's going on around you, but most of us move through our days seeing little past a morass of assumptions, projections, and preconceptions that lodged themselves in our field of vision a long time ago and have been collecting cobwebs ever since. Our eyes no longer serve us because we've forgotten how to see or judge anything clearly. When we lose our clarity of vision, our minds are no longer our own and we forfeit our powers of discernment. This is how we come to rely on dubious external authorities to guide us. Achieving inner clarity is a fundamental step to reclaiming our youthfulness.

Rejuvenate the Mind

If you wish to promote youthful vitality, you must become energetically whole again. Loosening the clutches of your ego—that part of you held hostage to social mores and expectations—and harmonizing your mental state with more-natural rhythms is fundamental to self-revitalization. Otherwise, any mental chaos and negativity will continue to imprint destructively upon you, upon your actions, and upon every cell in your body. This is the first barrier between you and what you want.

There are plenty of ways to begin lifting your subconscious and unconscious imprintings. I recommend finding a method that speaks to you. For example, you might begin by working with spiritual teachers such as Almine, Anita Briggs, and Guy Finley. There are many inspiring audios, videos, books, guided meditations, and recapitulation exercises available online, or you can choose to pursue some other method of removing the inner barriers to your clarity. (For recommended resources, visit the Forever Beautiful Shopping Guide at the end of this book and DetoxTheWorld.com online.) There are many methods of working the dissonance out. A combination of them have worked best for me. The only prerequisites are that you:

- see the value of a clear, calm mind;

- earnestly want to harmonize your energies;

- understand that it doesn't happen overnight;

- are ready to release old programs of regret, judgment, and victim-hood; and

- are willing to take personal responsibility for your present and future choices.

In my professional opinion, mental wellness is as important to the body's health as is blood chemistry. The typical modern person today is deeply polluted, with the mind's destructive patterns constantly reinforcing irrational consumption, chemical addiction, and personal disempowerment. As long as you're in the grip of this vicious cycle, there's no possibility of wellness, let alone true beauty and youthfulness. For the blood to be clean (which we'll discuss further in later chapters), it needs to be alkaline, bathed in life's vital essences—not contaminated by septic obstruction. The same goes for the mind.

A calm, clear, balanced mind is integral to clean blood and swift metabolic functioning because mental harmony supports mindful consumption and prevents mindless behaviors. One cannot have cells brimming with vitality and a mind cluttered with negativity. So stop squandering what mental energy you have left on life-sapping perceptions, thoughts, and value systems. These will only lead you to dangerous behaviors. Whatever is left of your life force is worth protecting—even if, like most people, you've spent your life letting it slip like sand through your fingers. As long as you still have a small spark of self-sovereignty left, you can work to reclaim your powers of perception.

Beware—Illusions for Sale

Everywhere you look there's a lie, a trap that can't wait to profit from your mental programming. It demands that you measure yourself against it. If you listen closely, you may even hear the sound of it sucking you in, convincing you that you're lacking something.

Here's what you must know: You already have everything you need within you.

Stop looking for the answers in cleverly packaged products. While there are some brilliant beauty enhancers on the market, it takes a discerning eye to parse out the naturopathic winners from the synthetic impostors, and these select items are effective only insofar as you stop blocking your internal wellsprings of self-regeneration. You have a zillion points in your body and in your energy field that link up with nature's larger matrix of life. You can get as much as you need from that matrix if you learn how to sync up with it. Life comes only from life.

Society has programmed you from birth to respond to certain ideas and images in predictable ways, defining your values at a very early age and reinforcing them throughout the rest of your life. Whether it is a quality, a look, a material possession, an evoked experience, a status, or some combination of these, our consumer culture is busy manufacturing and selling it to you every moment of every day. Yes, I freely admit, even this book that you hold in your hands—although full of much honest intention—is packaged and marketed to appeal to your social programming. Unless we live completely off the grid, we are all, to greater or lesser degrees, servants of the consumer market.

The question then becomes, for each and every one of us: What has become of my authentic self? It is still there? Was it ever? If so, how do I reconnect with it?

Until you learn to see clearly, you will be a sucker for every commercial image and ideology. Notice your reactions to the market-driven images around you. Are you always measuring yourself against them? Do they make you feel inadequate? Do they routinely convince you to buy the products they are selling—often at considerable financial and personal expense? How much of what you're buying, and *buying into,* is actually keeping you youthful, beautiful, and strong?

Embrace Change

This might seem obvious to you, but one of the biggest obstacles for people who want to change their lives is that they don't actually want to change themselves. They may think they do, but deep down the idea of it frightens them. They'd rather see the world change around them. Real change, however, must come from within. Sadly, most people spend their whole lives in a rut, fearing change. But living with the same mind-set, the same way of seeing, the same way of doing things, day after day, is barely living at all. It's your ticket to stagnation, calcification, premature decay.

Ask yourself this about every single thing you think, do, communicate, ingest, and buy: *Does this harmonize with nature's great living matrix, and does it help reconnect me with it?* If the answer is no, it's time to examine why you are buying into it. Be very honest with yourself. The answer may simply be that it's a social habit, or you like it, or you're addicted to it. Fine. It's your decision to make. But take responsibility for your decision. When you feel the prick of consequence later, instead of beating yourself up for it, or blaming others, let that experience inform your next decision.

The secret to changing yourself is changing what you value, not what you merely say you value or are told to value. For example, you cannot change from living in the past to living in the present until you come to value the present moment above all else. How do you do this? Usually, it takes an uncomfortable jolt of recognition (perhaps after one too many drinks, or a wasteful purchase, or a hurtful comment) to realize you're just skimming the surface of your life; that you are letting the present moment slip away, again and again, without ever really connecting with it; that you're missing out on your own joy and vitality. Worse, you may suddenly realize you are digging your own grave.

It's much easier to appreciate the present moment when you see it as your bridge to a better life. I urge you to give it the value it deserves. Let the pain of every misstep inform your next step. Try to be fully present in the moment and see where it leads. See what fruits you harvest when those little seeds—your little affirmations of life—grow into mighty trees.

This brings us back to the core law that teaches us to discern between what opposes nature and what harmonizes with it; what is real, living, and revitalizing versus what is illusory, lifeless, and devitalizing. Recognizing the difference, and then acting on that recognition, is your ticket to freedom—to your authentic self. Adopting the principle of clarity will ensure that you:

- choose to consume living substances over dead, devitalized ones;

- devote precious time and energy to what you actually value, not waste it on what our consumer culture convinces you to value; and

- reconnect with the natural world and come to recognize your authentic self, which has been there all along—often silenced but yearning to be heard!

Evolution by Co-creation

If you are going to practice the principle of clarity, keep in mind that there are as many ways of living as there are people on Earth. Each person sees the world uniquely, thereby creating a world that resonates with him or her. When you combine the many worlds made up of many people's visions, you create a collective reality—or a collective consciousness. However, this presents a chicken-or-the-egg conundrum, because while the collective is shaped by the way the individuals perceive the world, their perceptions hatch from a world that they inherit. So what each of us sees, although we are each unique, is a blend of inherited perception and unique perception.

Are you still with me?

Good!

Now, in an ideal world, this phenomenon would be a helpful tool in moving humankind forward. We would be evolving by co-creation. But this is assuming that we all learned to see clearly, to value life above all. The problem is that today, there are more barriers to clarity than ever before. Where we could be using advances in technology, medicine, and communications to serve our evolution, we are being completely outpaced, outsmarted, and oppressed by them—so that most of us can barely make heads or tails out of this blizzard of market-driven misinformation. We rely more than ever on others to shape our reality, to tell us what to buy or not to buy, to tell us what we must do in this busy, fast-paced world to be young, beautiful, successful, and relevant.

But young, beautiful, successful, and relevant to whom? By what standards? Who's calling the shots here? Personally, I have no interest in remaining youthful or relevant if it means systematically killing off life and perpetuating an unsustainable course. On the other hand, I recognize that the best thing about such a course is that it's unsustainable. That's fine. Let that world end. It won't be the end of the world—just the end of one that hasn't worked so well. If it were a machine being replaced by one that worked better, everyone would rejoice. Try seeing it this way and you'll relax. Releasing that world of devitalizing illusions, desires, insecurities, and fears can only serve you well. Stop trying to jockey for a position in it. Try opening your eyes instead.

Once we learn to see with our own eyes, to discern between corrupt marketplace illusions of youth, beauty, and power and the real things, we can apply the principle of clarity to every moment, thought, and action. Yes, every waking second, we can choose to break free of the tyranny of false values and re-create everything from the cellular integrity of our bodies to the world of life that we inhabit. Take a minute to consider the magnitude of that freedom. Yes, your thoughts drive every choice you make, every moment that leads to the next moment, and so on. So how do you want to use that freedom? Can you imagine effecting your own personal evolution, and, by extension, the evolution of humankind?

Seven Steps to Clarity

Step 1: Acknowledge your consumer values. Acknowledge that "mother culture" has had your ear from day one and take an honest look at all the nonliving things you have been programmed to value. What are they? (For example: cars, houses, clothing, jewelry, cosmetics, cereals, energy drinks, TV shows, celebrity gossip sites . . . the list is endless!) For clues, look around your home, your closets, your cabinets, your favorite Internet sites. Can you recognize these things as proxies for what your heart truly desires (e.g., security, self-confidence, beauty, youthfulness, love, laughter, energy, a sense of connection) and how widely most of them miss the mark?

Step 2: Travel down memory lane to the source of those values. Go back to your earliest memories and, from there, create a timeline of the popular cultural messages you received that taught you what was of value. How, or from whom, did you receive them? It may be helpful to break the timeline down into age brackets—i.e., 0–5, 6–11, 12–17, 18–25, etc. Trace your feelings back to the most vivid images and impressions that became the value directives in your life. (For example, it might be the feeling of joy when you opened up your first Barbie doll on Christmas morning; behind that were all the commercials that made Barbie the most important item on your "Dear Santa" list, and predetermined your concept of feminine beauty.) Now, who has been selling these impressions to you all these years? Pull the curtain back and take a good look at who or what is standing behind it.

Step 3: Recognize the patterns and behaviors that spring from those values. Take a look at your daily planner, weekly commitments, and monthly bank statement to determine how much of your time, money, and energy are spent on consuming nonessential products or else striving to be able to consume them. How much lasting satisfaction and fulfillment do those things bring you? How much disappointment, shame, or emptiness? Which ones make you feel your best and serve your greatest good? Which drain your energy and resources but seem like requirements for fitting in?

Step 4: Identify the present-day vampires that prey on your energy. Look at all the elements of your life that suck you dry. It could be the corporate job you hate but stick with because it pays for your posh lifestyle. It could be a relationship that has grown stagnant or is emotionally draining. It could be the high heels and the push-up bras that squeeze and angle your body in painful ways. Or the teeth whiteners, hair dyes, expensive lotions, and cosmetics that deplete your cellular integrity as well as your bank account. Or all the coffee and alcohol you consume daily to wind yourself up and down, up and down, so you can continue chasing after illusions of youth, beauty, power, and joy without ever quite attaining them.

Step 5: Mentally enter the stores you frequent and look at what they are selling. Notice how in any drugstore, grocery store, or department store, most of what they are selling is an illusion, pressing the buttons of your cultural programming. Notice how the stores themselves undermine your well-being with their unnatural lighting, chemical scents, blown-up images, sales offers, and blaring pop music—all to stimulate you to buy, buy, buy. More, more, more. Now, now, now. Notice how these stores prey on your well-known cultivated weaknesses. Do you only go into them for what you need, or do you often find yourself popping in for just a few items and emerging with a whole armload of well-packaged promises? How often do you fall into the compulsive shopping trap? How much waste and accumulation builds up in your home as a result? How does the psychology of shopping block your clarity?

Step 6: Envision a new you. You've just done the hard part—the honest assessment. Now it's time for the fun part—creating your vision. Imagine all the time, energy, and resources you could redirect away from wasteful consumption toward your regeneration. Envision yourself linking up with the natural world instead of constantly opposing it. Envision choosing only the most natural products, substances, and environments. Imagine not needing all the things the world says you need and making your own decisions. Imagine loving and honoring yourself as you might love and honor a child, a garden, or a work of art. Imagine what authentic beauty and youthfulness would look and feel like. Go ahead; close your eyes and envision it. Envision the you that would emerge once you've cleared away the cultural barriers and energetic vampires standing between you and what your heart truly wants. Imagine how light and free and energetic you would feel. Imagine the uplift of a clear, self-possessed mind, lit up with the most life-affirming values.

Step 7: Commit to that vision. You've seen the folly, you've identified its origins, you recognize that it only leads to decay, not to mention bankruptcy. And you've envisioned another way, another you. Now that you have your vision, it's time to commit to it. One by one, hold all of your thoughts and actions against that vision, and watch yourself—indeed, your whole world—unfold anew. Just put your feet on the bridge and start walking, shedding the old values and habits with each step. Keep moving until you get down to the real, radiant, irreducible you.

2. THE PRINCIPLE OF CONDUCTIVITY

The greatest measure of life is energy, and energy must be allowed to flow freely. Just as our thoughts cannot flow freely, clearly, and efficiently in a cluttered mind, energy cannot flow in an obstructed body. Where blockages occur, stagnation and calcification—the initial phases of the deterioration cycle—immediately set in. In order to prevent stagnation and calcification, you need to be aware of your blockages: where they are, how they were formed, and how to remove them.

Understanding Energy Patterns

If you could see the flow of your energy, you would see a pattern that looks like a giant elongated donut—a tube torus. Energy enters the vacuum of your north and south poles propelled by magnetic forces, and exits the poles propelled by radiant forces. This is how energy is constantly regenerating in a healthy toroidal field—in particular, in the human body, but more generally in cells and atoms, as well as in planets and solar systems. This toroidal field is the blueprint for all life as we know it.

Within this tube torus you have many energetic centers, from the larger chakra spheres to the subtler nadis, best known as acupuncture points. Your energy field lies within greater energy fields. What looks like empty space around your body holds a vast network of energy that enters your personal field, runs through you and back out again. Everyone operates within this vast energy matrix. These energy exchanges are occurring all around and within us, conducting throughout all life. When this energy flows freely, conducting vitality throughout the macro- and microcosmic toroidal fields, life thrives. It is when blockages occur—when energetic conduction is impeded—that imbalances and decay ensue.

Thus, all life is interconnected by a massive unseen network of pulsating energy—what I've come to call "source energy." You could liken the network to an enormous musical instrument carrying sound vibrations from its origin of creation throughout the whole pulsating apparatus. Or you might call to mind the ancient "music of the spheres" concept, which was used to describe the graceful, intertwined motions of the sun, moon, planets, and stars. Any way we look at it, whether we're talking about the individual cells within our bodies, our bodies themselves, or the great cosmos that we inhabit, we are all a part of this larger energy pattern.

This energy is not just vitalizing; it also carries information that directs our DNA. So as it recharges us, it is simultaneously sharing what's occurring in our environment with us, and we are sharing what's occurring within our cells with it. This continual intimate exchange informs our evolution, both in our lifetimes and across the generations. Our physical systems and their channels (e.g., vascular, nervous, endocrine, and digestive) echo our energetic patterns (meridians, nadis, chakras, and our toroidal energy fields). Wherever we go in the world—deep into the atom or out into the vastness of space—we find similar patterns, and it's by linking up with them that we can experience ongoing regeneration. We just need to learn how to plug ourselves into nature's vast energy network and activate flow!

As you apply the principle of conductivity to your life, don't be surprised if your mind gets sharper and your heart seems to expand as your body surges with new life. The resonant frequency of the "source energy" flowing throughout the natural world is manifest in the most incredible forms—in plants, animals, gems, metals, and so on. Masaru Emoto, a doctor of alternative medicine, popularized the notion that physical expressions are determined by the frequencies around them. Specifically, Masaru studied how readily water molecules reshape themselves according to surrounding vibrations. As organisms comprised mostly of water, we can expect our cells and physical systems to morph according to the frequencies we tap into.

Yet, we still routinely surround ourselves with dissonance and radiation—frequencies that threaten the integrity of our cells and systems rather than strengthen and beautify them. Meanwhile, we seek to rectify the damage with unnatural external substances and invasive treatments. To activate youth regeneration, we must find ways to bathe ourselves in the most harmonious environments, thus seizing the opportunity to absorb harmonious frequencies and reflect their beauty.

Cellular Cleansing

The most efficacious way to encourage conductivity in the body is to restore the body to an unblocked state. This is the purpose of cellular cleansing, otherwise referred to as deep-tissue cleansing. We begin applying the principle of conductivity on the cellular level because blocked cells make up blocked tissues, which make up blocked organs, which make up a blocked organism. The most proactive way to cleanse is to hydrate and magnetize waste residues up and out of the cells with water-containing, alkaline foods—namely, organically procured raw fruits and vegetables and their juices.

Most people have no idea how much impacted waste is lining the tissues of their organs. If they could see it, they would likely do everything in their power to remove it, especially if they realized that the waste was decaying them from within. The body is like a giant filter, trying to gather and expel anything that isn't for its highest good. But as the rubbish of unfit substances (in the form of corrupted food, drink, medication, air, water, and radiation) is constantly being forced into the body, it cannot excrete the waste through the eliminative organs fast enough. Over the course of decades of carrying around an overburdened filter, residue builds up in the cells, in the tissues of the intestine, and in other organs. If you are brave enough to stand the thought, you will accept the fact that you are saturated with this inorganic waste that is impacted like dry tar inside your body, creating multiple blockages in your system and prematurely aging you.

There is wonderful news, though. That "tar" can be removed, and you can reverse this accumulation through a twofold "awaken and release" method. But restoring conductivity requires dedication to a cleansing lifestyle and vigilant choices and behaviors, in order to (a) prevent further accumulation of waste and more blockages as you remove the old ones, and (b) maintain a freely conducting system. If you want to experience real transformation, all blockages in all parts of your physical and energetic bodies must be dissolved.

If you thought life was boring, try increasing your conductivity and you'll never think so again! You may have a lot of obstructions to dissolve. I did. It took me the better part of ten years to clear up my pathways for optimal conductivity. But every blockage I dissolved was worth its weight in freedom, and I could enjoy the process of self-liberation every step of the way. I never said this was quick and easy—only that it works a whole lot better than anything you'll find within the anti-aging marketplace!

Removing obstructions is infinitely more effective than slathering on "hope in a jar," because most products just clog up your cells and accelerate aging. Just start applying this principle, and you'll see results. The further you go, the more apparent the regeneration will be. You have a lot of cells in your body—trillions upon trillions. Make some headway on those cells and it will show.

The practical applications recommended below will help you to remove the blockages of stagnant matter and its by-products to reverse the calcification and decay that is decomposing your body from the inside out. This must be done for regeneration to occur when the body is in decomposition mode, which it typically is by your third decade of life—that's right, around age twenty-five! You'll be using the "awaken and release" method to magnetize, hydrate, and eliminate these blockages through your colon and skin as outlined below. As you do so, your liver, kidneys, spleen, pancreas, lungs, and lymphatic system will also be detoxifying and moving these blockages out. Talk about spring cleaning!

Awaken and Release

If you are new to cellular cleansing, do not to rush into eating exclusively raw, highly vitalized foods unless you plan on doing a great deal of colon cleansing right out of the gate. Simply introduce more and more of them gradually. Pure, organic, high-water-content raw fruits and vegetables are potent awakeners. They awaken the deeply embedded accumulated matter in the cells and tissues of the intestines, which is great if your body can fully eliminate all that is awakened by them. Most people cannot because they have overloaded bowels, and trying to expel the old matter is like trying to get a square peg through a round hole.

It may be hard to believe, but believe it: There is far, far, far more waste in your body than you can imagine—way more than you will expel in the first few days, weeks, and even months of tissue cleansing. The accumulation is epic, even if you are only in your twenties or thirties. Even if you have been a vegan, vegetarian, or otherwise conscious eater. Even if you appear relatively thin.

Non-water-containing foods are acidic, and acidic foods stick like glue in the system. While foods such as whole grains, organic chicken, non-GMO soy foods, legumes, and even organic dairy might seem like "health foods," I can assure you that they only make a partial exit after digestion because they are dehydrated, inflammatory, mucus-forming, and sticky—their positive ionic charge magnetically seals them to the negatively charged cells and tissues in the body.

Face it, folks, we've been eating many of the wrong things even when we thought we were eating well! Blame it on the misguided messages of our culture. We have been so cut off from nature for so long that we've lost our natural intuition about what's healthy and unhealthy. We've been letting health-food marketers direct our choices. The sad fact is, formula is not good for babies, grain is not good for humans, and even much of our produce is unfit for ideal human consumption.

We are beginning to dissolve the health and diet manifestos of our predecessors, but we cannot evolve fast enough culturally to prevent unnecessary deterioration. So if I were you, I would get wise quick to the realities of our times. This means to accept that (a) there is a huge amount of waste inside you; (b) the awakeners are water-containing, organically grown raw fruits, vegetables, and their juices; and (c) what may seem like too much deep-tissue cleansing is probably just cracking the surface of your toxicity.

If you face up to the facts and take swift action, you will begin to regenerate from within. If you drag your feet, I'm sorry to say, you will spiral deeper into deterioration and squander any opportunity to reverse course. Life is life. I didn't make up the rules; I am just the "minuteman" delivering the message because the enemy (premature aging, rapid decomposition, undignified death) is headed to your camp unless you shift course dramatically.

In practice, this means, first and foremost, that we must eradicate the blocks developed from our accumulation of waste matter and its by-products. I write about this extensively in my previous books, but to paraphrase here: Awaken + Release = Life Force Energy! The awaken-and-release method is the tried-and-true approach to tissue cleansing, and it's the cornerstone of my practice. It is fail-safe and powerful. You simply *awaken* the waste that saturates the tissues by hydrating and magnetizing it out of the cells with a diet very high in alkaline, organic, raw vegetable juices and raw salads. If you are new to this method, be sure to include some cooked vegetables and perhaps some less cleansing foods that you enjoy to avoid overburdening your system all at once. Then, with the help of properly administered enemas and colonics, you can *release* the awakened waste through bowel eliminations.

The longer you practice the awaken-and-release method, the more you will open up your body's pathways to conductivity. I recommend committing to at least three months of cellular cleansing to appreciate the profundity of the transformation—not just for a youthful appearance, but also for weight loss, increased energy, and mood enhancement. Most of my clients who commit to this initial period of experimentation find the method so rewarding and the accompanying lifestyle so enjoyable that they adopt tissue cleansing as a long-term practice.

Eating for Youthful Conductivity

Imagine a world where everything is alive—a planet of thriving rain forests, pristine mountains and valleys, and clean oceans. Imagine our world before it became littered with steel, concrete, plastics, and carbon monoxide. Now zoom in on the plants, soil, animals, insects, air, and water. Notice how every living element and organism draws its sustenance from its surroundings, both immediate and global; how they all take in and release electromagnetic energy from the sun.

We humans are no different. We, too, belong to this great ecosystem. We, too, are designed to conduct pure energy throughout our tissues, organs, blood, lymph, and neurological pathways. We, too, are a part of this wondrous, pulsating network of natural energy. The greatest folly of the modern diet is the idea that dense substances—animal flesh, grains, beans, processed foods, vitamin and mineral supplements, etc.—are what sustains us, when really it's living electromagnetic energy.

Imagine your body unadulterated by offensive substances, discordant frequencies, disturbed thoughts, and stressed emotions. Imagine your pathways and cells clean and highly functional. Imagine your mind surging with creativity, your heart filled with reverence for all life. Imagine taking only what you need, and always giving back. Can you envision it? Because this is the essence of youthfulness—a clear, ringing state of conductivity. This is you as a sustainable, interconnected being, one who honors all of natural life as you honor your own cells.

Eating for timeless beauty means taking in living foods—substances that themselves conduct energy. But here we must recall a critical caveat: Due to generations of clogging up the cells and pathways of the human body, we must first reverse the cumulative damage before we can partake of this exciting life-generating opportunity. But the most rarefied, high-frequency substances must be gradually introduced to the body while the system is being cleansed—most efficaciously through colonics and deep sweats. A diet of living foods can elevate the electromagnetic quantity and quality of the whole human system, if introduced gradually to an obstructed system.

Eating for conductivity is a whole new way to engage with food. Going beyond detoxing and cleansing, it is what comes once detox is accomplished. Food takes on new meaning. No longer is food about mere caloric and nutritional value, but about creating and sustaining a life-generating current, full of "force from the source." Once you are mentally and emotionally ready for this approach, plugging into a more life force–conducting diet will be a luxury, a pleasure. It will not cause suffering or a sense of denial because you will be in sync with a higher frequency, and this frequency will recognize the indulgence and appeal of water-containing, high-vibration foods. It's what your body has been yearning for all along!

When I was a little girl, I remember hearing my elders say that when a woman got older, either her face or her bottom would fall. The reasoning was that if she got a bit plumper, she could keep a more-youthful-looking face, but at the expense of her body; if she got skinny, she'd have a trim body but an old, sagging face. In fact, it seems to remain the conventional wisdom that older people either go to fat or get skinny and frail.

But when you understand the laws of natural electromagnetic conductivity and fully apply it to your body, you find that there is no differentiation between a youthful face and a youthful body. You can be youthfully lean with a smooth, youthful face when you eat living, energy-conducting foods, because the indwelling life manifests in the whole body. So eating for beauty and youthfulness means choosing the most vital plant foods. Among these are juicy tree fruits, because they draw their sustenance most directly from sunlight, but all fruits and vegetables are powerful alkaline agents for dislodging acid waste from the body.

Ask yourself, "What is the most beautiful thing I can consume today, or in my next meal?" A truly beautiful meal will be made of the purest substances you can find. This will be a very individual choice. For you it might mean a piece of organic fresh fish on a bed of heirloom tomatoes and lettuces; or, a baked yam with ghee and Himalayan sea salt served with homemade guacamole and carrots from your local co-op. Or it may mean an all-raw, water-containing, vegetable-based meal such as a blended green soup and massaged kale salad dressed with lemon-lime juice, stevia, and stone-pressed olive oil. Whatever the case, make it an opportunity to elevate your being. Remember: The foods you eat imprint energetically on your cells and tissues, and the best foods support the dissolution of blockages, reconnecting you with life's energy matrix. That is how the cleansing lifestyle can be an agent of transfiguration!

Raw vs. Cooked Foods

While you'll find some cooked dishes and even a few dishes with eggs and fish in the recipe section of this book, please note that these items are used as a transition tool to enable your body to start releasing accumulation from decades of nonideal eating. These foods are youth-regenerating only insofar as they enable you to initiate and commit to the process of cleansing. If you seek the highest levels of youth regeneration, eventually you will want to stop consuming animal products and cooked foods, at least most of the time, and adopt a 90 to 100 percent raw, plant-based diet. However, this all depends on your goals. The recipe section in this book includes cooked foods to serve as an excellent transitional bridge for the novice detoxer. If you are a veteran cleanser seeking optimum rejuvenation, move toward a 90 to 100 percent raw-food diet by substituting raw options for the cooked-meal options in the Three-Week Age-Defying Detox Plan. You'll find a lot more all-raw recipes in my previous books, particularly in The Raw Food Detox Diet, Raw Food Life Force Energy, *and* The Fresh Energy Cookbook.

Deep Breathing

The lungs are a powerful eliminative organ. Deep breathing not only floods the body with fresh oxygen and alkaline air with each inhale, but it also aids the detoxification process with each exhale. Children are naturals at deep breathing; notice how their bellies move in and out with each breath. Most adults, however, take short and shallow breaths. With deep, belly-centered breathing we can bring in more oxygen, and alkalize our systems with increased cellular respiration, releasing carbonic acid wastes from our cells. (Consider the fact that the longest-living animals on the planet, such as sea turtles and snakes, breathe deeply and slowly: a powerful lesson in breathing for longevity!)

It is also important to note that in times of stress, we humans shorten and quicken our breathing significantly. This is why consciously taking deep, full breaths sends the opposite message to our brain cells and helps to instill a lasting calm. Find time throughout the day to focus on breathing and reap the rewards of an alkaline body that is centered and relaxed. Let your belly expand on the inhale and contract on the exhale; if it helps, imagine drawing your belly button all the way in toward your spine on the exhale. Deep breaths massage the organs and clean the blood—particularly if you are exposed to pristine outdoor air. Pause occasionally during the day to notice how you're breathing and whether you need to make a conscious adjustment.

Deep Sweating and Sunbathing

Sweating helps to purge toxins and clear out blockages through the skin. Saunas, particularly the infrared variety, are useful for this. I use my infrared sauna every day except in summer, when I sunbathe frequently. If you don't have access to a sauna, you can get your sweat on through sunbathing and exercise.

Many people shun the sun completely. While it is wise to be vigilant about skin cancer and premature wrinkling, we should remember that the sun is a great healer and magnetizer—it can help pull toxicity out of the body like a magnet, the way green vegetable juice magnetizes acidic waste up and out of intestinal tissue. And yes, as we all now know, it's also very important for vitamin D!

However, our thinning ozone makes the sun's rays extremely powerful, so only expose your skin in the safe hours from dawn until about 10:30 or 11:00 a.m. or after 4:00 p.m.—depending on how strong the sun is where you are, how much melanin you have in your skin, and how obstructed your system is. Barring none, everyone I know who cleanses has corroborated that they do not burn in the sun the way they did pre-cleanse. Personally, I use the sun as a fundamental health tool, and spend as much time as my schedule will allow basking in the sun in the spring and summer!

I recommend avoiding putting any chemicals on your skin when you are therapeutically sunbathing. I firmly believe that the chemicals in mainstream sunscreens are carcinogenic; they go straight into the bloodstream and, when hit by the sun's rays, may create cellular abnormalities and mutations. You can wait another several years for all the scientific studies to corroborate this, but do you really want to do that before you stop slathering chemical creams all over your skin?

Pure coconut oil is the only substance I apply to my skin to keep it hydrated in the sun. I know that sounds crazy, but I generally only sunbathe during the safe sun hours, and I never burn, even when I sneak in some midday summer sun. I certainly burned before I started cleansing. What's more, I'm of Russian-Irish descent, with a naturally fair complexion! I suggest shading your face, neck, and décolletage with a hat after exposing it for just a few minutes in the direct light. Use your intuition and self-knowledge. Only you know the appropriate amount of sunbathing that will generate therapeutic results for you; but make no mistake, the sun is your friend, and the electromagnetic source of all life on this planet. And don't forget that the skin, your largest organ, can be a great eliminative organ when shedding toxicity.

A good dose of daily exercise should also provide a good sweat. While I am a big fan of yoga and of sweating, I am not a fan of doing yoga in a room heated with conventional heaters. If you wish to do hot yoga or Bikram, I recommend doing it in the summer in a shaded place or in a studio that has infrared heaters. Avoid breathing acidic air at all costs, particularly when you are breathing as deeply as required during yoga.

Deep Stretching

The next tool to prevent calcification and increase conductivity is deep stretching. It may seem simplistic at first, but don't let that fool you. As the great yogis have said, a person is only as old as his spine. If your spine is like that of a child, you are physically as youthful as a child. So stretch out the stiffness from your muscles and joints and increase your flexibility. You don't have to do yoga if you prefer calisthenics, but if you are not already an expert in correct alignment—how to bend, flex, and reach in ways that support your body's flexibility—you will need to learn from an experienced guide.

Increasing flexibility requires daily practice, but it only requires five or so minutes each day to maintain. In order to become flexible, you must break through blockages and dissolve them. Dissolving these blockages will open you up physically, emotionally, mentally, and spiritually. If you approach it with a positive, healing mind-set—as in, *I'm here to increase my flow and flexibility*, not *I'm here to get a yoga body*—deep stretching is extremely powerful. Just five minutes of it can help to open up your whole day.

Remembering the old adage that you're only as old as your spine is flexible, focus on stretches that emphasize finding your center. Here are three of my favorite deep stretches for increasing conductivity:

Spinal Twist

1. Lie on the floor on your back with your knees up and your feet planted firmly on the floor. Move your feet in toward your center as far as you can while still keeping them flat on the floor.

2. Allow your knees to fall to the right, stacking them on top of each other as much as you are able.

3. Let your head fall to the left, and stretch the left arm out on the floor in the opposite direction from the legs to allow the spine a deep, twisting stretch. Relax every muscle and lie in this position for one minute, then repeat on the other side.

Spinal Curl

1. Start in a standing position with your toes facing forward and your feet hip's width apart. Let your arms hang down naturally at your sides.

2. Imagining that the crown of your head has grown very heavy, allow your chin to begin tucking under as your head starts to pull down toward the floor.

3. Let the weight of your head continue to pull downward and slowly roll down along the front of your body until your spine is completely bent over. (Do this very, very slowly, one vertebra at a time.) Keeping your knees slightly bent and your arms hanging heavy, remain in this position for up to a minute, until you feel adequately stretched.

4. Then reverse the roll very slowly, straightening the base of the spine, the middle, the top, and then the neck until you are standing fully erect. Repeat this exercise three times.

Sitting Spinal Curl

Just as you gently reached your arms toward your feet and guided your crown toward your feet in the spinal curl, do the same but from a seated position, with your legs stretched out in front of you. I like to do this exercise in the bath when my body is warm and supple. It helps me to release any trapped energy in my spine and hamstrings for greater chi flow throughout the body. In a hot bath, you can enjoy a deeper stretch. If you are able, hold the stretch a little longer than usual; enjoy the deeper release and feel any stress dissolve into the water.

Rebounding and Whole-Body Movement

You want to increase the conductivity of *all* your pathways by exercising your whole body. Physical motion is a great way to break up stagnation, release blockages, and increase overall conductivity. It's also a natural way to kick the bowels into high gear, ensuring that you have regular, deep-cleansing movements.

I like rebounding best because it moves every single cell at once in a beneficial, low-impact way, massaging all the organs and animating the internal pathways and the internal waste systems. Biking and hiking in the open air are also great. Dancing is another great choice because it engages every body part at once, and releases so many nonphysical blockages in the expression of the movement. It's great for reconnecting with your body, increasing flexibility, and developing physical intuition.

One of the most youth-regenerating forms of exercise is jumping on a rebounder, a mini trampoline that provides nonimpact aerobic exercise. If you choose to buy a rebounder for your home, make sure it's a good-quality one. The bungee-cord models are best, but there are also a couple of excellent spring-based models (see the Forever Beautiful Shopping Guide). If you are fragile or do not have very good balance, you can purchase a bar for your rebounder to stabilize you as you bounce.

Jumping on your rebounder fifteen to twenty minutes a day will activate your lymph glands and develop beautiful muscle tone. Besides, it's fun! Put on your favorite music and jump around like a kid. In my personal and professional experience, I have found that rebounding as part of a regular self-care regimen helps to bring a tight, springy tonality to tissues and cells. A few things to know before you begin:

- Do not wear socks or shoes. Socks can be slippery. Shoes will wear your rebounder down unnecessarily, and deny your feet the natural reflexology treatment you get when you bounce. Bare feet are perfect!

- Always take care to rebound on an empty stomach, not after a heavy meal or large juice or smoothie. First thing in the morning or three to four hours after a well-combined meal is ideal.

- Start with just a few minutes and work up to a longer workout. Even if you are a veteran aerobic athlete, rebounding exercises all systems of the body, especially the lymph, which is not very clean in most people prior to cleansing. It also packs a wallop of an exercise punch. Some studies suggest that ten minutes on the rebounder is equal to thirty minutes of jogging.

- Finally, if you are a beginner or feel less confident about your strength and balance, you don't need to bounce so much that your feet leave the surface. Start with just bouncing gently. That alone will do wonders to tone your muscles and initiate lymphatic cleansing in a gentle, safe way for anyone at any life stage. Allow yourself to get acclimated to this new way of moving, and soon you'll be jumping like a cheerleader!

> *Walking on Air*
> *For a great beginner's exercise, try marching in place, lifting one leg at a time while raising the opposite knee. This should feel basic and intuitive as you jump back and forth from leg to leg, with a high bouncing step, for five to ten minutes. If you are new to rebounding, start with a maximum of ten minutes, and gradually build up to longer periods over the course of several weeks. You don't need to bounce very high to get a great effect, so start low, and as you gain confidence, enjoy jumping higher and higher, just like a child!*

What I don't recommend are high-impact exercises, such as long-distance running on concrete sidewalks or streets. Running periodically on a track or on grass is okay. Running barefoot on a beach a little more frequently is fine. Long-distance running causes reverberations of impact through the body, potentially harming bone and weakening skin tissue, particularly when done on concrete. It's hard for people who love to run to accept this. Running is a go-to sport for high achievers and those looking for the best calorie- and stress-release bang for their buck. I can personally appreciate this; I ran for years. But running regularly very long distances on concrete is very much in opposition to nature, and the impact often shows on the gaunt, tired faces of runners.

While you may be tempted to focus on "trouble spots" when you exercise, I urge you to remember the value of whole-body movement. It is great for dissolving physical and emotional tensions. Tensions create blockages and calcification—the opposite of youthful conductivity. Let this, above all else, be your reason to exercise!

Dissolving Cellulite

Cellulite is one of the most common complaints among my private clients when they first come in to see me. By the same token, one of the benefits that most amazes them about cleansing is that it makes their cellulite disappear! The development of cellulite is governed by the following set of factors: diet, conductivity, hormone balance, toxicity, and water retention. People often think it's hereditary, but my personal and professional experience has proven otherwise.

Fundamentally, cellulite is caused by poor conductivity—an obstructed flow of life force through the body. Naturally, if your diet is dense with too much cooked and processed foods that are not well assimilated and eliminated by the body, intestinal and cellular stagnation will develop. Add to this stagnation the accumulation of environmental estrogens. Estrogen increases fat storage, and it also feeds yeast, triggering addiction to sugary, starchy foods. This in turn creates a vicious cycle of more harmful consumption, more fat storage, and further stagnation. Your final ingredient for cellulite is toxicity. The body is always trying to keep toxins away from the vital organs, and the safest place to store them is in the fatty tissue. So, the adipose (fat) tissue becomes a receptacle for toxicity.

Fluid retention increases the appearance of cellulite. The body retains fluid when we eat packaged foods or excessively salty or fatty foods. When these fluids combine with fat cells, the fatty tissue becomes more pronounced. Consuming a diet of mostly water-containing plant foods prevents water retention and, in fact, enables the body to release undesirable stores of stagnant fluid, dramatically reducing the appearance of cellulite.

The cycle of cellulite buildup will continue until all of the contributing factors are systematically rectified. Here is how it's done:

- Clean up the diet dramatically, focusing on greens and exclusively organic foods.

- Draw out waste accumulation through the bowels and skin.

- Rebalance the hormones.

Dissolving cellulite takes time as the body heals, but once the blood that feeds the cells is clean, oxygenated, and freely conducting, the cells and tissues will discard what is no longer needed, and eventually the body will be renewed without cellulite. In my opinion, this is a far superior method to liposuction—no cutting and sucking, just internal repair for lasting cellular transformation.

3. THE PRINCIPLE OF LIFE FORCE ENERGY

If you think having a fat bank account is desirable, try having all the trillions of cells in your body ringing with abundant life force. Your life force is not some imaginary sci-fi substance; it's a scientifically measurable electromagnetic current that animates your body. Whatever you choose to call it—vitality, life force, prana, chi—it is indeed a very real presence, and you are utterly dependent on it. To be youthful is to have an abundance of freely conducting life force. In light of this concept, take a moment to savor Chaucer's springtime imagery in *The Canterbury Tales*:

Whan that Aprill with his shoures soote
The droghte of March hath perced to the roote,
And bathed every veyne in swich licour
Of which vertu engendred is the flour . . .

There is no sweeter sensation than this coursing of youthful vitality, which springs eternal in the natural world. I have experienced this rush of vitality again and again within my own body, and it is the closest thing I have yet felt to immortality. When the blood and the mind are freely flowing and conducting the elixirs of life, they unite as a veritable fountain of youth. As lushly as the flowers and the foliage of spring, we humans can also spring anew!

Once you honor the principle of conductivity and unblock your pathways, you can start to feel the real power of these little electron-energy spinners conducting from cell to cell, suffusing the blood, tissues, and organs. If you remain stagnant, in a state of decay and decomposition, they will flee the nonviable environment. This is what's happening when you lose your strength and energy: Your life force is leaving. You have to give it a reason to stay.

If you open up your pathways through detoxification and deep stretching, the electromagnetic party can begin, pulsating vitality throughout your whole body, sparking like the lights of a pinball machine—*bing, bing, bing!* Of course, to be clear, the atoms we want at the party are only those with a negative ionic charge; that is, those with more electrons spinning on the outer belt of the atom than there are protons in the nucleus. Atoms with a positive ionic charge will steal and neutralize atoms with extra electrons— they are the electron party crashers!

When we recognize that our bodies are pure life force energy, then we can appreciate that the only means of caring for ourselves is to promote that energy in our bodies every way we can. Cells must be vitally suffused with chi from plenty of negatively charged atoms. Elasticity in cells and skin tissue depends on this subatomic charge. The most effective strategy for getting electrons to the party is to open up the pathways, per the principle of conductivity, and then to aggregate electron power from outside sources. To discover what those sources are, read on.

Eating for Life Force

The foods you eat, the liquids you drink, the air you breathe, and any supplements, medications, or other drugs you ingest all must go under critical investigation. If you are taking a medication, it is because you are out of balance. In almost every case, the question to ask is not "Should I take the medication?," but "Can I remove what's causing the imbalance?"

Do you live mostly indoors eating devitalized foods, locked in codependent relationships that isolate you from the larger community? Are you always thinking about the past or the future, with little concern for the present? If this describes you, you are not alone. Most of us lead disconnected lives, cut off from a world that could nourish us if we'd only let it in. Wherever you experience pain and imbalance you will find blockages and broken connections. Once these blockages are removed (most tangibly experienced through cleansing the pathways, cells, and tissues in the physical body) and these threads are reconnected, the presumably inevitable "symptoms of old age"—such as stiffness and joint pain, decreased energy, poor memory, insomnia, and a sluggish metabolism—will evaporate. If enough of us get wise to the facts of youth regeneration, our whole medical and health-care system will be forced to get wise with us.

The greatest living foods on the planet for humans are fresh, water-containing, organically grown fruits and vegetables and their juices. When properly grown, these foods are among the cleanest, purest life forms, drawing their own life force directly from the sun's energy. When you have a clear, freely conducting system and consume a diet of mostly organic, living foods, your life force energy quotient will rocket, and you will feel the difference in your whole body.

You will also *see* the difference. Life force is a harmonious frequency, which is a precursor to form (all energy is a precursor to form). Therefore, once your body is abundantly flowing with it, your physical appearance will transform to reflect its vitality and harmony. It will not just be an external facade! Every cell in your body will be thus transformed. So, yes, you will look fantastic on the outside, but you will also be glowing on the inside with vibrant blood cells, bouncy organs, and witty neurons firing accurate signals from brain to body while your endocrine system secretes its hormonal elixirs beautifully.

Water Content

Conventional wisdom tells us that we should drink eight glasses of water each day. This a classic issue of quantity versus quality. The question we really need to be asking ourselves is, What kind of hydration does the body need, and are we supplying it? Water is the quintessential superconductor. Life force is electromagnetic, so water is central to the functioning of our being. But isn't water, water? No, not by a long shot. First of all, water needs to be living to contribute to our optimal hydration.

Let's consider the quality of the soil in which our fruits and vegetables typically grow. This is not widely discussed, but it is critical. Had an inorganic carrot lately? Dry, flavorless cardboard, right? The typical farmed carrot

What about an All-Raw Diet?

I've underscored the importance of transitioning away from mainstream foods toward a mostly living foods in all of my books because that is the most effective way to support the cleansing process. But beyond this transition phase, an individual who has significantly tissue-cleansed might opt for a purely live diet. You will know you have reached this stage when, left to your druthers, you would naturally choose living foods for every meal. This is an elevated stage of youth regeneration: You awake each morning full of energy and optimism; you are symptom-free; and your bowels are strong and active enough to eliminate well daily—granting you a feeling of lightness you haven't felt since you were a child. If you get to this stage, I highly encourage you to go with your inclinations and not let social pressures and lifestyle obstacles hold you back.

I have gone through this process myself and find that while cooked foods had a place in my life for a long time, there came a time when even cooked vegetables and goat cheese undermined my higher harmonics. This is not the case at every stage, but if you persevere on the youth-regenerating path, you are likely to find yourself at this stage at some point. Know that it is an excellent place to be, but it is only a choice, not an end-all-be-all goal, and certainly not a command of the age-defying detox method.

carries less life force today due to dryer, devitalized soil. The water is coming through a pipe from some unknown source, being artificially recycled and treated with chemicals. This is not nature's fountain of youth. This method of agriculture may seem to work for a while because the power of life force starts out so strong that it takes time to witness its signs of degeneration. But once we start to notice the effects, it is already late in the game.

To keep your body properly hydrated with life force, remember the maxim "Drink your food and eat your water." By that I mean, drink your fresh vegetable juice, the most concentrated nutrition you can get, and eat a diet of mostly water-containing organic fruits and vegetables. If you are dutifully drinking eight glasses of water a day instead of consuming your daily greens and other water-rich vegetables and fruits, you are not getting the type of hydration you need to remain healthy and youthful. By contrast, if you enjoy nature's most hydrating foods and juices on a daily basis, you won't need to drink all those boring, flavorless glasses of water; you'll be getting most of the water you need from your food, and a powerful array of enzymes and nutrients besides!

All that said, drinking pure water is still essential for health. Whatever your water source, be sure it is absent of fluoride, chlorine, and bromide (i.e., avoid tap water whenever possible), which inhibit the thyroid, preventing hormone secretion and interfering with pineal gland function. In addition to drinking clean, living spring water, I highly recommend taking a unique and very specific form of iodine called "nascent iodine." Nascent iodine will help to chelate these chemicals from the body while supporting the reactivation of thyroid hormones. We will discuss this special supplement again in Part V when we talk about hormone replacement therapy and the thyroid.

Vitamins and Supplements

The term *supplement* implies that there is a deficiency to fill. So if we are thinking of taking supplements, the first question to ask ourselves is, Why is there a deficiency? The answer is most likely a combination of the following:

- Our dietary intake lacks the subtle and gross nutrients we need to sustain our cellular functions.

- Even if we are taking in an organic diet abundant in water-containing plant foods, the soil the produce is grown in is itself depleted of vital substances.

- Our bodies are so filled with impacted waste matter that even the best nutrients cannot adequately reach the cells and tissues that need them.

Waste accumulation is the most universal problem for every client I have ever had, so let's address that first. In my professional experience, before the waste is sufficiently cleared from the body, supplementation with anything other than vegetable juices and raw salads is useless. Once a significant amount of this obstruction is cleared by the awaken-and-release method, two seemingly miraculous things happen:

1. Life force flows and conducts more freely throughout the body, creating a palpable uptick in energy.

2. The body absorbs so much more of the vital essences from the raw juices and salads and is able to convert the various nutrients into the substances that it requires, thereby eliminating many of the initial deficiencies.

Simply put, cleansing empowers the body to create what it needs from the substances we give it. This is why cleansing, as a first step, is so much more effective than the common approach to nutritional supplementation, which only has us taking in more substances that our bodies are ill equipped to use. Remember, this dynamic system of nutritional synthesis has kept humans evolving for millions of years, long before there was any such thing as a vitamin shop!

Once we cleanse and rehabilitate the body's natural ability to use nutrients to serve its immediate needs, we can work on strengthening our various systems with selected vitamins, minerals, and chelators (supplements that help to remove environmental pollution and heavy metals). In a cleansed, realigned body with clear, conducting pathways, these supplements can work much more efficiently. They can get right into the cells and tissues and work their magic.

Vitamin and mineral supplementation can also be helpful after pregnancy and while nursing, particularly for mothers who undergo multiple pregnancies. Pregnancy can drain a woman of her personal mineral reserves and leach her thyroid hormones, leaving her with weak bones and teeth and a hypoactive thyroid (i.e., producing too little of the thyroid hormone). If the deficiencies aren't rectified immediately, her skeletal and endocrine systems will continue to weaken, making her more prone to energy loss, weight gain (fat storage and cellulite), and rapid aging. It's a snowball effect. This is why women who don't meet their nutritional needs during this delicate time typically find that this is when everything starts to fall apart for them, inside and out.

In our culture, pregnancy is the time when women are encouraged to eat whatever they want, giving themselves a nine-month license to indulge. However, it's during pregnancy and nursing that it's most important for a woman to be extra vigilant about taking in only pure, nutrient-rich foods. Given what we now know about cleansing, nutrition, and responsible supplementation, there is no need for women to degenerate from vixens to grannies overnight after pregnancy!

Detox for Immortality

Now that we've established that the cleaner your cells are, the more life force can flow through them, I'll share with you an intriguing experiment to ponder:

As described in his book, *Man, The Unknown,* French surgeon and Nobel Prize winner Dr. Alexis Carrel kept a chicken heart alive and reproducing new cells for twenty-eight years (chickens typically only live about eight years). His research indicated that he could have kept it alive indefinitely. All he did to create "immortal" conditions for this chicken heart was to keep the cells in perfect conditions—a saline solution that was the perfect temperature, pH, and nutrient-mineral balance—and ensured that the solution was immaculate every day by flushing any toxic wastes and acidic by-products. The cells did not die of aging; Dr. Carrel simply stopped the experiment. Thus, Dr. Carrel posited: "The cell is immortal. It is merely the fluid in which it floats which degenerates. Renew this fluid at intervals, give the cells what they require for nutrition and, as far as we know, the pulsation of life may go on forever."

So why do cells die and become cancerous or otherwise nonviable? Because the cells' fluids become toxic, operating against the natural flow of life force. Substances that are not intended for cellular health corrupt it. If they are flushed away, the cell has a chance at viability; as long as the fluid is clean, the cells have an untold life expectancy. When cleansed daily, the cells that make up our tissues and organs can ring with life force, and that is reflected in our overall appearance. Consider this as you consider the role that colonic irrigation plays in the age-defying detox method. Cleansing is a key priority here because not only does it ensure that the body is flushed of the causes of decay, but it is also the most expedient way to ensure the robust flow of life force.

Young Blood

When I started studying live blood microscopy and actually had the chance to see what pathogens such as fungus, bacteria, and viruses and their waste products do to healthy blood cells, it became clear to me that purifying the blood is absolutely fundamental to health and rejuvenation. To speak of youth regeneration is to speak of blood regeneration. Only clean blood, flowing to all the organs of the body, can give them the fresh nourishment they need for continual regeneration. Clean blood is vital, youthful, and free of pathogens; dirty blood circulates toxins and is a habitat for pathogens. Young blood is something we can enjoy at any age if we take the necessary steps to restore it—and this is precisely what the detox lifestyle is designed to do. I highly recommend hiring a distinguished live blood cell analyst such as Richard Harvey (whom I interview on page 167) to conduct a live blood cell analysis on your blood. It is powerful and empowering to see the state of your blood and the very real interactions taking place deep in your veins. It will motivate you to make the best daily choices for blood health and youthfulness like nothing else.

Fresh Alkaline Air

Take every opportunity to breathe in clean country or wilderness air, such as on mountains, in forests, and on pristine beaches. Even if it's just on weekends, once a month, or on holidays, every cleansing break from city pollution helps to bring in the life force. If you can't get out of the city for a long stretch of time, do the next best thing and go for brisk walks or bike rides in the park. But clean, alkaline wilderness air is so much more electromagnetically alive than urban or suburban air. Think of the air around you as the plasma that you swim in. You cannot expect to swim in acidic plasma day in and day out and embody the qualities of youthfulness. Indulge in clean outdoor air as often as possible.

4. THE PRINCIPLE OF GRAVITY AND LEVITY

So much of the aging process has to do with gravity—the constant downward tug on our physical features. But as living beings, we have the gift of levity to counterbalance gravity. How gravity affects us depends largely on the conductivity of the body's internal pathways. Gravity can be counteracted in many ways—for example, by improving circulation, practicing inversions, sleeping properly, and exercising positive thinking.

Just as there is a force of gravity weighing down on us at all times, there is the levity of the life force that is forever seeking to lift us up. This levity is what makes plants and trees reach toward the sunlight and enables countless living creatures to stand upright and leap into the air. In a world of dwindling life force and increased stress, fear, and disappointment—all accomplices to gravity—it's easy to get passively dragged down in body and spirit. It's all too easy to forget the levity within and around us that's just waiting to be tapped. So the first thing is to become aware of the force of levity, to imagine it brimming from every atom and every electron of every cell.

Try holding that image until you *feel* the levity. It's a distinct sensation. Go on, humor me. Take a moment to imagine a forest of trees in an utterly pristine region. I like to think of the cedars in Siberia (as vicariously traveled via the *Anastasia* book series). Imagine these pristine trees vibrating or "ringing" with life. Become one of the trees for a moment and imagine yourself ringing with life too. Allow the sensation to come. It should feel like being home—but home as your soul knows it. Hold the sensation and feel it intensify. You cannot see it or touch it, but it is undoubtedly real. As you "ring," feel the levity of your cells. They are not being pulled down but are buoyant in their cellular fluids. The more you exercise this awareness and shed the dissonance from your life by making choices that resonate with this sensation of levity, the more you will become that frequency, and your life will reflect it back to you.

New Age theorists typically use the term *ascension* as a way to escape the body and the material realm. There is a deep misperception among many religions that the material realm is lowly, and that to be redeemed one must ascend out of it. This is a shame. The forces of levity flow through everything, including matter. In the atoms that make up the molecules of material life are these amazing little beings called electrons, which can send out healing energy waves. They contain the energy of our bodies and the world around us just as drops of seawater are holograms of the sea. These electrons have levity, but if devitalized by common living, they cannot serve us. Clean, open, freely conducting pathways allow these electrons to carry the force of levity throughout one's whole being, raising one's cellular vibrations and preventing the organs, tissues, and body from succumbing to the force of gravity.

In addition to meditating on levity and adopting the attitudes that support it—such as love, praise, forgiveness, and gratitude—there are other practical ways to exercise levity. Read on.

Sleep for Levity

Here's a simple tip: Sleep flat on your back. We have made sleeping very complicated with lots of pillows, but the best way to sleep is with the spine totally flat, without a pillow. Babies and small children almost always prefer to sleep this way naturally, which is why you'll often find them in the morning sprawled on their backs, with their arms outstretched over their heads.

Part of the problem is that people typically go to bed too full to lie perfectly flat, especially if they experience acid reflux. You will not experience this problem if your evening meal was a reasonable size, well combined, and given enough time to move through the stomach and reach the intestine. If your midsection is calm, you will be able to lie comfortably flat on your back. If you really love pillows, use a soft, squishy one under your head— one that gives you a little prop but not so much that your spine is misaligned and your face is slanted and prone to the tug of gravity.

Don't believe it'll make a difference? Try it. Sleep flat on your back for eight to nine hours each night and notice the difference in your facial skin, in the integrity of your back, and in your circulation.

Also, be sure to get enough sleep each night. Ample sleep has never been more important than it is today. The modern world is awash in acidity, from chemically processed substances, polluted air and water, high levels of personal and professional stress, and radiation from technology. Sleep is the time when you metabolize (i.e., digest, assimilate, and eliminate) all that has entered your system during the day so you can be clear for the next day. If you do not clear out yesterday's debris, you will increasingly weigh yourself down with the burden of toxic accumulation. This is why people are typically stinky when they get up in the morning. The body is employing all its various tools to "clean house." It's only when you're not eating or running around that your body can start to process the accumulated waste.

Sleep is often talked about (usually in the context of not getting enough of it) and universally regarded as important, yet it is often neglected in daily life. Without the naturally cleansing, healing aid of a good night's sleep, you will compound the effects of gravity and accelerate the aging process. Sleep is a great agent of youth, and far more powerful than many people realize. Create a sleep routine and honor it. Your whole body will thank you for it, and will work all the more efficiently as a result. We will discuss sleep further in Part V (see page 139).

Alcohol, Gravity's Accomplice

I highly recommend reducing your alcohol intake as much as possible. Today we are exposed to way too many toxins, acidic substances, and agents of decomposition. We must strive to cut way, way down on exposure to these degenerating substances. We have to process whatever we're exposed to, and exposing ourselves to more than we can process is a fast track to deterioration (i.e., premature aging and sickness). Also, the more we expose ourselves to gravity's accomplices—and remember, alcohol is a depressant that will drag us down mentally and physically in the long run—the more we need to sleep to help fight them off and regenerate energy for the next day. Think about this before you reach for that next glass of wine or bag of junk food.

In the past I have formulated transition diets that permit the occasional glass of wine, and wine has been one of my personal indulgences, but I would like to clarify that wine is not conducive to beauty and youthfulness any more than beer or hard liquor is. While wine can be a helpful transition tool, enabling a beginner or intermediate cleanser to enjoy familiar social experiences, it acidifies the blood and interferes with circadian cycles and organ regeneration.

Do not fall for the seductive marketing that suggests that wine is good or natural for you—it is not! All alcohol is acidic and yeast-feeding, just like chocolate and grain. Nothing acidic and yeast-feeding qualifies as a health food. Enjoy them if you like, but don't be fooled into thinking they are going to do your blood chemistry any favors. The antioxidant and anti-inflammatory properties heralded in red wine actually come from the resveratrol in red grape skins, not from the alcohol. So enjoy organic red grapes, sans the acidic alcohol quotient.

For many years I continued to enjoy wine guiltlessly; I believed I was "getting away with it," since everything else I did was so alkalinizing and life-generating. But eventually I had to face the fact that I was deceiving myself—that the wine was poisoning my internal terrain. The acidic, fermented substance was enabling bacteria, mold, and fungus to thrive in my bloodstream. It was also interfering with deep sleep and robbing my organs of the full benefits of nightly regeneration. It took me a long time to accept this because I loved my wine. I still enjoy it, but not nearly as often. As a result, I sleep much more soundly and deeply, and I don't get as dehydrated.

Alcohol and Dehydration

Because alcohol is so acidic, the kidneys go right to work trying to neutralize the damage it is doing and flushing out the toxins as quickly as possible by forcing urination. Alcohol also interferes with the production of a hormone produced by the pituitary gland called ADH, which regulates urination. This all leads to increased urination and dehydration, which is very aging indeed!

Like cigarettes and coffee, alcohol does not appeal to one who isn't addicted to it on some level. Take a break from imbibing for even two weeks, then notice how strong and acidic, perhaps even off-putting, the alcohol tastes. This is the same reaction your tender cells have to the substance. It makes them recoil and feeds the rogue bacteria in your body.

Since wine has a high sugar content in addition to being acidic, when you stop drinking you may experience strong cravings for starches and sweets. This is because the yeasts you have been feeding with wine are looking for food. If you can avoid feeding these yeasts with other sugars or starches at this juncture, the yeasts will eventually starve and stop bothering you for food. Be strong and focus on the wonderful alkaline plant foods you can enjoy, including fresh organic fruits, raw treats, and the addition of a few drops of stevia instead of sugar.

If you do wish to enjoy wine on occasion, 1) make it a rare indulgence; 2) be sure that everything else you take in is alkaline; 3) take wheatgrass juice for three consecutive days following the alcohol intake. This will give your body the support it needs to prevent your internal terrain from succumbing to the proliferation of rogue bacteria and fungus. The important thing is to be honest with yourself and take responsibility for the choices you make.

Youth-Regenerating Refreshments

To help cut back on your alcohol intake, treat yourself to delicious, visually appealing refreshments instead. Make a carafe of purified water flavored with lemon, orange slices, and mint. Or you might prefer cucumber slices with dill or basil. Young coconut water and iced herbal tea are also delicious options that are great for gatherings and parties. Get creative; indulge your taste buds. Just remember that nonalcoholic sparkling wines are just sugar and carbonation, so don't fall into that trap. All carbonated drinks are acidifying and wreak havoc on digestion and bone health. The goal is to flood the body with oxygen and to expel carbon dioxide.

Inversions

All of your pathways and organs benefit from practicing inversions, which simply means lying straight and flat on an incline with your head below your feet. You can increase the intensity and effect of the position until you reach a full vertical inversion (aka, a headstand or a handstand). This, however, is not necessary to reap the health benefits of inversions. In fact, for most people, especially those who are overweight or symptomatic, full vertical inversions are not even recommended. Nothing is gained by inverting more than what the body is truly ready for.

For most people, I recommend gentle inversions on a body slant board. A body slant board elevates the feet about eighteen inches off the ground. An inversion board, by contrast, allows you to manipulate the grade of the inversion. However, the eighteen-inch inversion is so beneficial at all stages of regeneration that you may never want or need more than that. Even though I will often practice a full vertical inversion, I still use my slant board daily. I find gentle inversions more relaxing, and I can spend more time with them; my organs benefit from the lift and change of direction, increasing circulation and oxygenation. Perhaps best of all, using my slant board allows me to refresh my perspective and calm my mind and body. If I am feeling out of balance, I simply lie on the slant board for a few minutes and feel immediately rebalanced. I can greet the rest of the day with fresh vision.

If you don't want to purchase a slant board or an inversion board for your home, you can build your own, or just use a sit-up bench in your gym. Choose whatever method works best for you and your routine. Reversing gravity this way is extremely beneficial—not only for the face-lift it gives you, but also for the way it lifts your internal organs, taking the weight off them and giving them a chance to breathe, change direction, and circulate blood, chi, and lymph. Just remember, whether you are sitting, sleeping, standing, or lying in an inverted position with your feet above your head, proper alignment is intrinsic to optimal flow and conductivity.

Make sure you only invert on an empty stomach. I recommend inverting before eating or drinking anything, so that it's the first exercise you do upon rising. Otherwise, you may practice inversions several hours after eating a properly combined meal. Note that gas rises when you do an inversion, so it may help you to release trapped gas! (For more information about inversions, see page 111.)

Skin Care

The integrity of your facial tissue depends a great deal on the interior state of your body, but in addition it requires a unique care regimen. Find a simple cleanser and moisturizer that work for your skin and use them consistently. Use only the purest products. For cleansing, I recommend either organic all-natural soap or a cleansing milk. After cleansing the skin, immediately apply a powerful moisturizer. I personally prefer oils to creams. I used to have combination skin, but thanks to the detox lifestyle, my skin is no longer dry or oily but balanced and healthy.

The seasons may affect your regimen. For example, you may wish to reapply facial oil often during the dry winter months and less often during the sticky summer months, as I do, but keep in mind that skin likes consistency. Find what works for you; don't treat your skin like an experimental canvas for all the latest products and fads.

Keeping maturing skin juicy and moist is important to image-conscious youth-seekers because well-hydrated skin will not hold wrinkles. I know that many people are concerned that oils will clog their skin, but in my experience that is only true for mineral oils and oils with unnatural ingredients in them. In conjunction with tissue cleansing, which decreases acne-causing bacteria that moves through the blood and tissues to the skin, clean oils have a predictably favorable effect. If you do not practice tissue cleansing, I cannot make you any promises. If you do, oils will become your skin's best friend! If you have some breakouts as you're cleansing, take heart—it is temporary; if you persevere, you will remove the cause. Of course, you'll want to take care not to introduce bacteria topically to your skin, but keep in mind that the majority of acne breakouts begin inside the body.

If you wear makeup often, be very careful with your application and removal. It's essential to keep the skin well lubricated. Be sure to apply a lubricant before you apply makeup; this will allow the makeup to glide on easily, without having to tug at the skin. I find that coconut oil is the best natural eye makeup remover.

If you use clogging, toxic products and exercise poor hygiene, then you can expect to have breakouts and other skin irritations. It's also natural to break out during PMS or when you've consumed more toxic substances than usual. Whether you're a teenager or pushing forty, a mainstream lifestyle will make you prone to acne. Find a good aesthetician to remove bacterial blockages and clogging, especially if you live in an acidic city environment. Get your skin professionally cleaned by a skilled aesthetician, and then make the effort to maintain it. *Never* go to bed with your makeup on. Think of cleansing and moisturizing your face each night as a sacred ritual. Use whatever routine works best for your skin, but in most instances it should only take about three minutes to go through the entire process.

While I don't believe in using a lot of products, there are several brands that I respect—in particular, Living Libations, The Body Deli, and select products by Decléor and Fresh. In the Forever Beautiful Shopping Guide I provide a list of my favorite brands and products; they are all made with the most natural ingredients. The same is true for any makeup I use. While I enjoy beautifully developed products just as I appreciate an inspired salad or raw dessert, I don't need them to be fussy. Just as carrots, apples, and bananas are perfect as they are, coconut oil, vitamin E oil, argan oil, and rose oil are fuss-free beauty supporters all by themselves.

Makeup Detox

This would be an ideal time to clean out your old cosmetics and upgrade your selection with more detox-conscious brands to prevent introducing dangerous toxins into your bloodstream topically. Also, if possible, try to go a few days a week without wearing makeup. This will let your skin rest and breathe free. If you feel you can't, or if you work in an environment that demands makeup, find other ways to rest and regenerate your skin. For example, you might take a soothing bath and coat your face and body with argan or coconut oil after work, or go for a long walk in the fresh air. Look for opportunities to offset the acidity and stress of your work environment. Every little bit of relief helps.

Vanity

At first blush, the detox approach to timeless beauty may appear to be linked with vanity, but it is most powerful when we focus on expressing our authentic nature rather than impressing others with our external image. To illustrate this bit of wisdom, let me share two stories with you.

When I marvel at my mother's youthful face, she sometimes reminds me of a story she read when she was reading a book on Christian Science by its founder, Mary Baker Eddy, called *Science and Health with Key to the Scriptures*. The story originally comes from an English magazine, *The Lancet*. It's about a young woman: Disappointed in love in her early years, she became insane and lost all account of time. Believing that she was still living in the same hour which parted her from her lover, taking no note of years, she stood daily before the window and waited for his return. In this mental state she remained young. Having no consciousness of time, she literally grew no older. Some American travelers saw her when she was seventy-four, and supposed her to be a young woman. She had no care-lined face, no wrinkles or gray hair; youth sat gently on cheek and brow. Asked to guess her age, those unacquainted with her history conjectured that she must be under twenty.

Granted, this young woman had a serious case of arrested development. We don't want to live lives of delusion! The point is that in her mind she was young, and so she remained effortlessly youthful. Time need not have the hold on us that we presume it must have. Remember the great proverb, "As a man thinketh in his heart, so is he."

Let's juxtapose that tale with another that many of us know well, Oscar Wilde's *The Picture of Dorian Gray*. Like the fate of Narcissus, who falls so in love with his own reflection that he dies staring at the image he could never interact with, Dorian Gray's ugly demise begins with his legendary vanity. When an artist makes Gray his muse and paints his portrait, Gray, finding fulfillment of the external senses to be the only thing in life worth pursuing, chooses to sell his very soul to ensure that his beauty will never fade. As Gray pursues a hedonistic, decadent, self-centered life, the portrait captures his true essence. Although Gray does not age, his portrait ages and grows disfigured, revealing the effect that each of his selfish acts has had upon his soul.

The moral of both stories? As you apply the principle of gravity and levity to keep your body as vital as possible, remember the natural law "as above; so below"—and, I would add, "as within; so without." Your body will radiate health and beauty insofar as your cells and your soul are filled with health and beauty. Avoid the trap of focusing too intently on your exterior, which will only lead to self-degenerating choices. Obsessing about your external appearance will cause you to neglect your internal terrain. By focusing on a life of compassionate connection, by embracing humanity and actively participating in the beautiful network of life, you will feed your own beauty.

A great runner doesn't stop to admire his stride as he races. An eagle doesn't stop to glance pridefully at his reflection as he soars. The pleasure is in the soaring; the success is in the act. The greatest gravity-defier is authenticity. So check your vanity at the door and regenerate youth for the sake of life—*all life*.

5. THE PRINCIPLE OF RITUAL

Everyone loves a brilliant idea. Most people's ears prick up at the potential of tapping into their own greatness. In my practice, I've seen hearts surge with excitement and relief to discover these principles of timeless beauty. But if someone leads you to good, clean, revitalizing water, that person cannot drink it for you. The question is, Are you going to drink deeply of this new knowledge? Will you put the principles into practice?

These principles are powerless unless you take them to heart and put them to task. It helps to ritualize these principles into a practical lifestyle. I can assure you that anyone who has accomplished anything of note has attained it through ritual—consistent, dedicated practice as a fundamental and soul-satisfying imperative in their daily life. The biggest block is usually an excuse that one perceives as immovable, such as the demands of long work hours or childrearing. But, as the saying goes, where there's a will there's a way, and ritualizing principles into practice is the most effective way of weaving them into the fabric of your life. This is far more effective than trying to heap them heavy-handedly on top of all the responsibilities you already have.

The effects of these principles and practices are cumulative and most dramatic when applied in concert. The whole is much, much more than the sum of its parts. These practices bring balance and harmony to every cell and system in the body. But it's up to you to create the rituals.

Expect your age-defying beauty ritual to evolve. What you start out with today will flow and change because you will be flowing and changing with it. Your rituals will become more connected and intuitive, whereas at first it may have seemed a bit forced. For example, you might start out just rebounding or stretching more, but then you might find that sleeping flat also makes more sense. Then you might find you've grown tired of expending energy on certain practices or products you no longer believe in—any of the countless absurdities of modern life that keep us on a short leash. In growing more aware of that leash, you will become emboldened to cut it, to set yourself free.

My own personal-care rituals have evolved a great deal over the years, molding with my family life, my discoveries, and my growing intuition. At times, I've learned the hard way why I cannot afford to neglect my rituals. I gauge my life now by my inner connectivity. I am always getting better at reading myself and adjusting my rituals accordingly. When I have fewer demands, I require fewer rituals. When life is running at high speeds, requiring a high level of output, I need to engage my rituals to the max in order to remain centered and energized. In the latter scenario, I design my rituals with great awareness and self-respect so I can neutralize all the energy-sapping demands.

Removing stagnant energy is a daily task, and absolutely essential for rejuvenation. Anything degrading to nature that we absorb must be released. Living in opposition to nature is the fundamental cause of aging and disease, and while it is impossible to eradicate all unnatural elements from life in the modern world, there is much we can do to peel back the layers of toxic accumulation, increase conductivity and life force, and infuse levity into every aspect of our lives.

As you come to learn the language of your body, you'll develop effective rituals and unite them seamlessly with your life; eventually, you'll practice them as naturally as brushing your teeth. At first, you'll build them into your life deliberately, working them around your schedule, but then there will come a beautiful tipping point when your life becomes a natural expression and extension of these principles. It may take a while or it may happen quickly, but as you awaken to the regenerating effects of these practices and principles, you will intuitively want to remove obstructions and stagnant energy and practice levity whenever possible. The very concepts of diet and exercise will change in your mind, and like a child you will rediscover the natural joy of movement.

As you become more vigilant about those aspects of your life that leach energy and make your mind chaotic, you will seek release from them. You will find that with each absurd program you release, you'll feel a surge of power and self-sovereignty. You will stop trading in your authentic self for a manufactured idea of what you should be. You'll fully appreciate the power of youth regeneration, feeling no need to defend your perspective or practices to anyone at any time. You will experience an uplift in body, mind, and spirit unlike anything you'll find at a doctor's office, and people will begin asking what you're doing differently to get that youthful glow.

Best of all, instead of having to admit to (or lie about) all the surgeries, drugs, and cosmetics you've resorted to, you will be happy to tell them the truth, just as I've told you. The principles and practices of timeless beauty are not for the privileged few. As living, breathing, self-renewing creatures of energy and light, lasting youthfulness is our birthright. It's just a matter of honoring its principles as we circle the sun, year after glorious year!

Morning Routine

The moment you awake, before you even get out of bed in the morning or say anything to anyone, breathe deeply, yawn, and stretch your limbs luxuriantly like a cat. If you haven't gotten enough sleep, or if you feel devitalized from indulging in too much food or drink the night before, think about how you will make these insults up to your body. Visualize the day ahead and what you hope to accomplish. Just as you have a ritual of brushing your teeth, taking a shower, and getting dressed, you can fashion a ritual of waking that will set you on a positive trajectory for the rest of your day.

Note that when you wake up in the morning, your body will communicate many things to you if you pay attention. Learn how to read the signs. If you overate the night before or did not sleep properly, you may look older than usual. When you're undergoing a detox, however, you might look awful in the morning, with fluids retained around your eyes and cheeks. If this is due to detoxing, don't despair—it's just the awakening of waste through the body. The lymph is cleansing, and on the other side of the cleanse you'll wake up glowing and youthful. If you commit to clean living, awakening to a beautiful face can be an everyday experience.

Meditation

While seekers of mainstream anti-aging solutions are busy spinning their wheels—or, as I like to call it, running their energy—age-defying detox adepts rest often and deeply. Meditation is a proven method of rejuvenation and increased mental health. Mental chaos always shows in the body and face. A quiet, clear mind is essential for sound decision-making and conducting life force. Build time for meditation breaks in your schedule, and clear the decks for it whenever you feel unexpectedly imbalanced. When you breathe, be sure your whole body breathes. Look where your thoughts and beliefs and energies are leading you, and think about where you really want to go. It may take only a few minutes of deep, meditative breathing to reorganize your energy, or it may take longer. Eventually, it will come naturally to you as a centering part of your daily life.

There are many different approaches to meditation and various guided meditations available on the market. Among these, I highly recommend those that enable you to reach the most youth-regenerating "delta" and "theta" level states. One of my favorite practices is delta-wave meditations. Delta waves are associated with the deepest levels of sleep; an hour of delta-wave meditation can renew the body like an extra sleep battery. That is not to say it can take the place of a deep night's sleep, but entering delta-level consciousness during the day will help to regenerate you. Theta levels, which are associated with meditation and light sleep, are also very restorative.

For excellent delta- and theta-wave meditations, I recommend those created by Anita Briggs. You can find them on her website (innermasterytools.com), or on my website (detoxtheworld.com). These meditations are between forty-five to sixty minutes in length, and can carry you into states of profound regeneration. You will feel your cells buzzing with vitality when you "come to" after one of these unique meditations.

Play

Remember the quote from *The Shining:* "All work and no play makes Jack a dull boy"? Well, it also gives him a dull old-man complexion! Why drag your feet when you could be bouncing or floating through your days? Bring back a sense of fun and wonder. Throw down a mat for some spontaneous stretching, open the windows to your stuffy office, take a music break, move your body. Such revitalizing actions hardly take any time, and can do wonders for your quality of life. (And remember, we all wear the quality of our lives on our faces, as clear as day!)

Make a space for community and learning from others. If you have children or work with them, observe the way they move so freely and with unself-conscious joy, and let them revive the inner child in you. Make a regular "play date" with a friend or family member. Go on a walk, pack a picnic, toss a Frisbee! Playing—setting your mind and body free—even for short bursts of time, will boost your youthfulness, creativity, and productivity.

Spa Treatments to Avoid

You can do more to revivify yourself at home with the right knowledge and access to colon hydrotherapy than you can do at even the best spas. But what if you want to go to a spa? What treatments are useful and which are not? The simple answer: You can tell which ones are useful if they result in revving up the lymphatic system, aiding waste removal from the body, and increasing chi throughout the body's systems. Below, I list specific treatments that support youth regeneration, but first let's take stock of those treatments that do not.

Certain treatments work directly against the natural processes of the body, triggering cycles of unnatural decay, which only necessitate further unnatural treatments to maintain appearances. Many of these treatments expose your skin and bloodstream to harmful chemicals, synthetically manufactured ingredients, and animal products.

If you are serious about rejuvenation, stay away from the following treatments:

Injectables

These work in two ways: either to impair muscle function (like Botox), or to fill hollow or lined areas of the skin, such as sunken cheeks or thin lips (fillers like Restylane and collagen).

Although they can't help with excess sagging skin, soft tissue fillers can add more volume and provide immediate results at a lower cost than surgery. These are usually Juvaderm or Restylane, a non-animal-sourced hyaluronic acid. The visible benefits of these treatment are temporary, and thus must be repeated and maintained, which means they are gradually absorbed in the bloodstream and in the body at large. Silicone oil injections, which build up over time instead of being reabsorbed, have not been approved for use as tissue fillers in the United States but are sometimes used "off-label" (not as indicated by the FDA or the manufacturer).

These dermal fillers are often used in conjunction with other "skin rejuvenation" treatments, such as injections of botulinum toxin, which freezes the facial muscles that pull on the skin and create lines and wrinkles. Botox comes from a bacteria that is a type of botulism. Botulism is found in spoiled beef and can cause you to get very sick if ingested. The word *Botox* is a combination of botulism and toxin.

Crystal Microdermabrasion

Crystal microdermabrasion is the traditional type of microdermabrasion which uses fine crystals to smooth and abrade the skin. The shredded dead cells, dirt, and crystal residues are then pulled away to clean and exfoliate the skin. This type of microdermabrasion uses chemical crystals such as aluminum oxide, sodium bicarbonate, sodium chloride, and magnesium oxide. The most commonly used abrasive crystal is aluminum oxide, which is known to be the second hardest mineral after diamonds. These crystals are questionably sourced or synthetically manufactured.

Chemical Peels

In this treatment, a chemical solution is applied to the skin, which makes it "blister" and eventually peel off. The reason this is so dangerous and potentially harmful is apparent in the name of the treatment. Before you get a chemical peel, your doctor may ask you to stop taking certain drugs and prepare your skin by using other medications, such as Retin-A or Renova. (The chemicals in these peels are intensive enough that they are known to interfere with medications and may necessitate more chemical use.) The doctor may also prescribe antibiotics or antiviral drugs. A variety of other toxic chemicals, such as phenol, are also used for deeper peels.

Implantation

Cutting the body open and inserting foreign matter opposes the age-defying detox method at the most fundamental level. Implants are used for everything from plumping cheeks and buttocks to augmenting breasts. Saline and silicone, the most commonly used implants in the United States, have the potential to rupture, create scar tissue in the surrounding area, and necessitate traumatic and heavily medicated surgery. They must also be replaced after their shelf life expires.

Spa Treatments to Embrace

The following spa treatments, on the other hand, complement a youth-regenerating lifestyle. They are noninvasive and naturally purifying and cleansing, benefiting the body as a whole.

Mud and Clay Treatments

Mud or clay baths as well as facial and body masks are a wonderful spa treatment option for detoxification through the skin. Uncontaminated earth and clay are alkaline substances that attract toxins and impurities, which will work their way out through the dermal layers and get absorbed in the mud. A mud or clay treatment will help to clear the pores and cleanse the lymphatic drainage system.

Colonics

More enlightened spas are starting to offer colon hydrotherapy along with other treatments. This is a promising development for the seeker of timeless beauty. One-stop shopping! Choose closed-system gravity-method treatments wherever possible.

Saunas

Infrared saunas provide an intense form of detox therapy. Infrared heat is a healing light frequency, which, unlike traditional saunas that merely heat the air and the surface of the body, penetrates five to seven centimeters into the body, encouraging a far deeper yet more comfortable sweat. This deeper sweat expunges far more toxicity through the skin than traditional saunas. Like traditional saunas, infrared saunas can be used daily by anyone who does not have high blood pressure or heart issues and isn't pregnant. Simply shower off afterward and a huge job has been completed.

In terms of duration, I generally recommend starting with fifteen to twenty minutes per session, which should encourage an initial sweat, and working up to a much deeper sweat that typically requires more like twenty to thirty minutes for most people. As your tolerance increases, you will be able to stay and sweat longer. Depending on how much time you have and how quickly your body responds to infrared heat, I would say anywhere from twenty minutes to an hour is appropriate, but never to exceed an hour.

Listen to your body and be sure to stay well hydrated with plenty of pure water during and after your sweat as needed. Other dry-heat sauna therapy is also effective as long as perspiration is produced, but nothing compares to infrared heat.

Ice Pools

Northern Europeans have been taking plunges into frozen bodies of water for hundreds of years, reporting marked improvement in one's complexion, immunity, and even libido. Many spas offer this option in conjunction with saunas. The contraction of the surface layers of blood vessels in the skin create an invigorating rush and leave your skin glowing. This is a great complement to heat therapy. It's really easy to get these benefits from hot-cold showers at home as well. Simply give yourself an icy rinse for a couple of minutes after your hot shower. Repeat the heat and cold again as desired.

Seaweed Wraps
Wrapping the body in chlorophyll- and iodine-rich sea plants not only nourishes the body through the skin (it's like being immersed in green juice!) but also magnetizes toxic impurities from it with its alkalinity. Skin becomes tighter and softer, and the body feels cleansed and deeply relaxed after a treatment.

Lymphatic Massage
The lymphatic system is a delicate yet strong and extremely important part of the waste-removal process in the body. This massage technique, which follows the direction of lymph flow throughout the body, is a very specific procedure. While it is surprisingly light-handed and gentle, it is also very pleasurable. The lymph is close to the surface, so don't expect a deep massage. Lymphatic massage aids detoxification by helping to unblock the lymphatic system, allowing the fluid to drain more effectively, restoring this critical internal cleansing support system to full strength. It can also alleviate fluid retention by opening these lymphatic pathways; many people notice a tighter, firmer post-massage result. The best spas typically have massage therapists trained in lymphatic massage, even if it's not listed on the spa menu.

Cupping
Cupping massage is an ancient Chinese and Russian healing modality used to increase the peripheral circulation of the blood, lymph, and interstitial fluid, thereby greatly improving metabolism and respiration of the skin. Cupping is highly recommended for the treatment of cellulite problem areas and is great for lymphatic facial massage. (For more on cupping, see page 81.)

Mineral Baths
Like mud and clay immersions, as well as seaweed wraps, alkaline mineral baths magnetize toxins out through the skin. They also soften and condition the skin, and provide a deep relaxation that helps to release muscle tightness.

Fruit Acid Peels

These peels use the natural glycolic acids from fruits such as oranges and apples to remove older layers of skin. There are several noted benefits associated with such a procedure, including improved skin tone and texture, because the acid penetrates the skin for a thorough cleansing action. This can help to prevent and fight acne. The acidity levels can vary from one product to another, so begin with a solution that has low acidity levels, and then gradually work up to solutions with higher acidity levels as necessary. Always seek a certified professional to administer this service.

Crystal-Free Microdermabrasion

Crystal-free microdermabrasion (or diamond peel) uses a diamond-tipped wand to provide skin abrasion and exfoliation. Unlike crystal microdermabrasion, this procedure does not use crystals to resurface the skin; instead, it uses a diamond-tip wand. This method works with the natural texture of the skin and does not cause the same trauma to the dermal layers because the wands are made specifically for different skin types and depths of resurfacing. Dead skin cells are vacuumed from the surface of the skin.

Oxygen Treatments

Many spas now include oxygen treatments, which let you breathe higher concentrations of oxygen, or have it infused through the skin in an oxygen facial. Oxygen therapy is a highly effective alternative medicine, just beginning to enter the medical spotlight. Its healing medical uses are employed in combination with vitamin infusions and essential oils in these spa treatments to achieve the same effect: regeneration and healing of the face and body through increased circulation, with a beautiful aesthetic result.

Beck Protocol (SOTA Instruments)

These products are available at home to follow the health protocol designed by physicist Bob Beck, who discovered a natural way to prompt the body to regenerate and heal while ridding itself of alien microbes. His protocol has not been the subject of medical research, but thousands of people have given testimonials of their results—everything from weight loss to remission from cancer. Beck created a three-part program for optimal health:

- *Blood Electrification through Micro-Pulsing:* This technique uses micro-currents to stimulate the body's use of natural electricity and to promote more energy and greater health.

- *Ionic Colloidal Silver:* Ingesting colloidal silver helps to promote healing in a natural, non-drug fashion.

- *Freshly Ozonated Water:* Drinking ozonated water oxygenates the blood, which may help to remove toxins, boost the immune system, and increase energy.

SOTA has created products that are widely recognized as the best Beck Protocol tools available. They sell a Protocol kit, along with instructions for use which vary according to the issues being addressed (www.sota.com).

Remember: The above spa activities are not mandatory for youth regeneration by any means. I have listed them to help you discern between life-generating and life-deteriorating treatments, so you don't waste time and resources on counterproductive services, and so you can indulge in supportive services when you desire them.

Wardrobe Upgrade

Throughout our lives, we go through several incarnations of styling. We begin with what our parents have us wear, then what our friends wear, then what celebrities and fashion icons wear, then what we think our romantic partners want us to wear, and what certain occupations, events, and various social conventions dictate that we wear. Let's face it: Dressing in the modern world is stressful. But it doesn't have to be. Here's what happens when you embrace the principles of timeless beauty:

- You naturally shed excess weight, so clothes start to look better on you in general.

- You stop acting like a marionette (always dressing for others) by loosening the strings of social conditioning.

- You clear away the clutter of your personal space, including your closet, to better reflect and support your clarity.

- You discover the fabrics and styles that makes you feel the most confident, comfortable, and authentically *yourself.*

It took me years to realize that I'm generally not a jeans and pants person; not only are they too constricting for me, but they don't flow well with my body shape. I feel my best in dresses and leggings. I've learned which shapes and textures I like most—hello, cotton and cashmere!—and which just bring me down no matter how much I like a styling concept in theory. Comfortable shoes are a critical part of a youth-regenerating wardrobe. I am not a heels person, yet I wore heels for more than two decades before accepting this about myself. I like riding boots, ballerina flats, and stylish sneakers. I only ever wear heels on rare occasions; I like to be able to move fast, and putting on heels is like putting brakes on my expression. But that's just me. Find out what's right for you.

Dressing is one of those things we do every day that can either put us in sync with our bodies and our spirits or in opposition to them. Give yourself the luxury of dressing in ways that make you feel as good on the outside as clean blood makes you feel on the inside!

Committing to morning rituals, meditations, play dates, spa treatments, and a wardrobe upgrade are just a few suggested ways to ritualize the age-defying detox principles and practices into your lifestyle. There are many, many more. I urge you to be creative but also honest about which ones will work for you. Each and every day, find ways to:

- Avoid calcification.

- Increase circulation.

- Promote flexibility.

- Remove distractions, chaos, and obstruction.

- Dissolve mental chatter through meditation and deep breathing.

- Counterbalance gravity with levity.

- Avoid toxic places and people.

- Maintain clean cells and a healthy intestine through an alkaline diet and cleansing methods.

- Sleep at least eight hours a night, or as long as you need to neutralize and metabolize all the acidity that you are exposed to during the day.

- Keep the mind and heart agile and light by releasing dogma, resentments, and other calcified modes of thinking (e.g., blame, criticism, self-loathing).

You might worry that ritualizing these youth-regenerating practices will make you high-maintenance. If so, keep in mind that you'll be clearing your schedule of all the old activities that have been running your energy dry, as well as all the old self-care rituals that have been prematurely aging you. You're dumping a huge load to take on a handful of activities that are going to make you feel feather-light!

RECAP OF THE PRINCIPLES

To recap, modern aging and disease is caused by living in opposition to nature. When you join forces with the powerful current of natural life force, you whole being responds and begins to regenerate from within. The five key principles of timeless beauty are:

1. **The Principle of Clarity:** This takes us back to the initial tenet that teaches us to identify what opposes nature and what does not. We must begin to discern between the two, if we are to lift ourselves up and out of a paradigm that opposes nature. Ultimately this is our ticket to freedom—not just to a more youthful appearance, but to all

of those enviable qualities that young people enjoy before they start colluding with the life-deteriorating paradigm.

2. **The Principle of Conductivity:** A healthy, youthful body is one in which energy is freely conducting. Where blockages occur, stagnation and calcification (the initial phases of the deterioration cycle) immediately set in. In order to prevent stagnation and calcification, we must be aware of our physical, mental, and emotional blockages as they occur, and work through them via various cleansing methods.

3. **The Principle of Life Force Energy:** This essential substance of life must be present in overflowing abundance. Life force is a measurable subatomic energy wave generated by rapidly moving electrons. Call it by any name you like, but life force energy is what animates us and continually revitalizes us. The purpose of increasing conductivity is to be able to conduct life force energy freely and abundantly. We can measure our youthfulness by the amount of life force flowing unobstructed throughout us day in and day out.

4. **The Principle of Gravity and Levity:** The force of gravity must be counterbalanced. The effect gravity has on us depends on the internal movements of the body—the rate of circulation and free-flowing life force energy. Gravity can also be counteracted by inversions, proper sleeping, reduced alcohol intake, stress release through meditation, and (as introduced in the following pages) facial exercises.

5. **The Principle of Ritual:** The principles of timeless beauty are only as valuable as they are practically applied to our lifestyle. Ritualizing the principles into daily practice is the most effective way to integrate them for lasting results. Through personalized rituals that are followed with dedication but that also adapt over time, we can reap the unlimited rewards of youth regeneration.

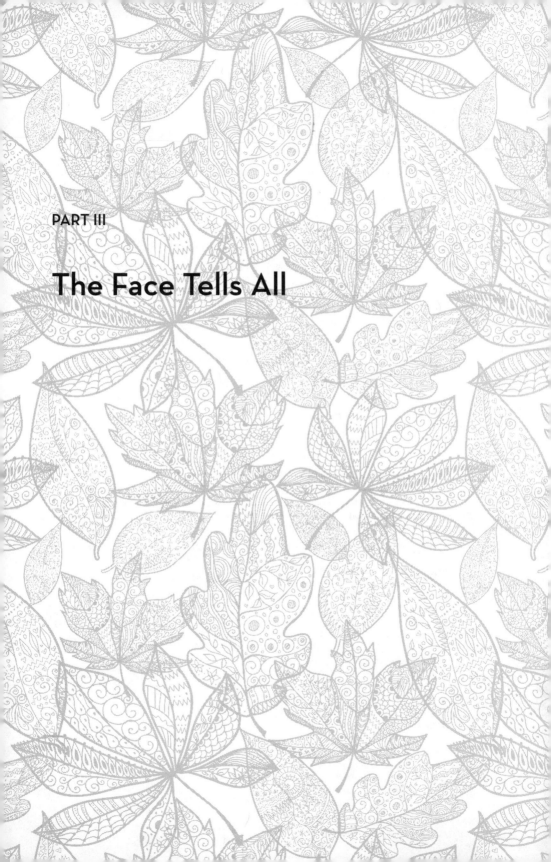

PART III

The Face Tells All

The face mirrors the interior state of the body, reflecting the condition of its cells, blood, and internal organs. It tells of cleanliness and filth, of harmony and discord, of wellness and disease. The eyes, too, are windows to the internal terrain. Studying the eyes for indications of bodily health and disease is called *iridology*. Studying the face is called *physiognomy*. The Greeks originally practiced physiognomy to read character in people's faces, but for our purposes here, we are interested in the quality of the skin and facial tissue for indications of poor health and premature aging throughout the body.

The face tells all if you've learned how to read it. When you mask the face through cosmetic facial treatments such as lasers, injections, and plastic surgery, you block this window to your internal health. So it is wise to become literate in the language of your face and body, and use that language to help you direct your life choices. A falling face reflects a devitalized body with cells, tissues, and organs that are not adequately receiving or conducting life force due to accumulating too much matter, toxicity, and stress. Here are some specific signs to watch out for:

- Weight and discoloration around the eyes and nose signal an overwhelmed liver and kidneys—too much animal protein, cooked fats, drugs, alcohol, or pharmaceuticals.

- Deep lines around the mouth and puffy lips indicate constipation and stomach problems.

- A yellow tinge to the whites of the eyes typically indicates liver disease.

- Bulging eyes raise the alarm that there is a serious thyroid imbalance, typically a hyperactive thyroid. This can be a sign of Graves' disease or goiter.

- Deep creases across the forehead and between the eyes also indicate liver and intestinal stress.

- Oily skin can either mean that there are too many fats in the diet or a hormonal imbalance due to the combined effects of diet and inherited toxicity.

- Oily breakouts, from fungus and bacteria, and sagging may indicate gallbladder and pancreatic stresses from imbalanced food choices and an excess of other unfit substances—particularly excessive starches and sugars, environmental estrogens, antibiotics, and hormones.

- Wrinkles and dry patches may indicate systemic dehydration.

- Blotchy red skin (particularly around the nose) often indicates too much alcohol intake.

In short, the face shows the degree of toxic accumulation or vitality of the organism. Vitality flows in an upward direction like a flame. When you see a downward droop to the face, what you are seeing is dwindling life force. As long as the skin is still thick enough in the first couple decades of life, before toxic accumulation has reached maximum capacity, it won't necessarily sag; but once that thickness dissolves, often noticeable by the late twenties and thirties, that face will start to fall.

The cells of your sensitive under-eye skin tissue will quickly reflect back to you the effects of your anti-energetic thoughts, behaviors, habits, and experiences—for example, the fact that you finished off the better part of a bottle of wine, or didn't sleep more than four hours the night before. Your face also reflects your environment, the energetic soup of your world, be it the miasma of street traffic, exhaust, and other city pollution or a messy home with domestic quarreling. Whatever it is, your face will reflect it, and no amount of foundation or cosmetic surgery will help. Living against nature and absorbing negative energies will cause you to lose your shine. Yes, you will lose that glow of youth before your time. What a thing to allow! I urge you to get hip to the red flags and protect yourself from the onslaught of negative energies.

NATURAL FACE-LIFT EXERCISES

Now, before you make the dire decision to undergo facial surgery, or to get Restylane or Botox injections (which are extremely toxic and degrade your blood chemistry, affecting the viability of every single cell in your body), consider this very exciting alternative method: natural facial restoration through muscle manipulation. Not unlike food combining and tissue cleansing, up until recently, this method of facial rejuvenation has been overlooked by the mainstream, and thus available only to those willing to seek out alternative paths. It's so simple and requires nothing other than a mirror and a few fingers—so simple, yet so effective!

This long-lost art of improving the integrity and appearance of facial skin through targeted exercise of the facial muscles is a brilliant option. I learned it from my mother, who learned it when she was immersing herself in the very avant-garde holistic health movement with Dr. Bernard Jensen and Dr. Gaylord Hauser in the 1960s. Today, at seventy-plus years young, she has a practically flawless face and outstanding muscular and skeletal integrity. She has incorporated these exercises into her beauty routine since her thirties, and I have not seen any other women her age with such a youthful face—and this includes those who've gotten face-lifts, cheek and lip injections, and chemical peels!

You can effectively transform your facial structure and restore levity to your gravity-prone face. The face is made up of muscles, just like your limbs and torso. However, facial muscle tissue is thin, which means it needs fewer repetitions of muscle contractions to be given a workout—just a few minutes a few times a week. You can do these while sitting, standing, or lying down. However, if you have access to an inversion board that you can place on a gentle incline, this will significantly enhance the effectiveness of these exercises. An incline helps to lighten the force of gravity and increase blood flow and oxygenation to the muscles. But with or without an inversion board, facial exercises work beautifully.

The following series of movements are designed to keep the facial muscles in peak condition, so that the face maintains its shape and taut appearance. To use these successfully, make them part of your daily routine. The first few times, try them while looking in the mirror, making sure that the way you engage the facial muscles is not contributing to wrinkles by unnecessarily creasing the skin. None of the following movements should create any creasing when you do them. If they do, simply place the fingertip on the creasing area to keep it smooth while you exercise. Once the muscles begin to feel fatigue, you can stop. The face is made up of small, delicate muscle groups that respond very quickly to small amounts of exercise. Straining them is not necessary. Repeat each movement only until you feel the burn. I hope you enjoy these facial exercises as much as I do!

The Gobble Gobble

As we age, the skin connecting the chin to the neck can begin to sag. This exercise targets the "turkey gobble" that develops when these muscles are underused and slack.

1. Stick your tongue out straight as far as it can go.

2. Curl your tongue up toward your nose while thrusting your lower jaw forward. Make it just a quick jab, then retract the tongue.

3. Repeat until you feel the muscles under your chin begin to fatigue (5 to 15 repetitions).

Starlet Eyes

This exercise has been affectionately nicknamed "The Renée Zellweger" for the way the actress lifts the apples of her cheeks toward her eyes when she laughs and smiles. It targets weakening and sagging skin underneath the eye (the "bags") and the top of the cheeks, which can hollow with age unless the muscle structure remains firm.

1. Open your eyes wide and stare at a fixed point in front of you.

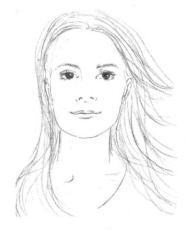

2. Slowly scrunch the lower lids as if beginning to squint, but without moving the upper lids (maintain the wide-eyed stare). The corners of the eye should not crinkle.

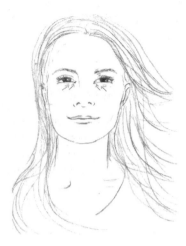

3. Open the eyes back up by releasing the slight squint and repeat until the under-eye area becomes fatigued (5 to 15 repetitions).

Pack Your Bags

The area directly beneath the eyes probably shows the biggest signs of aging, acidity, and organ fatigue. This movement will make you feel like the apples of your cheeks are popping up toward the lower eyelids. It will exercise and tone this area, encouraging fresh blood flow and firmness.

1. Thrust the tip of the tongue out and straight down toward the ground while opening the mouth as wide as possible.

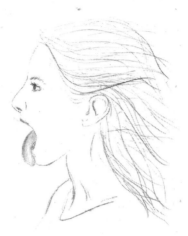

2. Retract the tongue and close the mouth. As in "The Gobble Gobble," this movement is just a quick jab.

3. Repeat this movement until the jaw muscles become fatigued (5 to 15 repetitions).

Forehead Push-ups

Don't forget the forehead muscles. If you keep them fit, they won't atrophy and be so prone to holding deep wrinkles. Forehead push-ups will tighten and tone this area so you don't have to wear bangs as you get older (unless you truly want to)!

1. Place two to three fingers horizontally across your forehead, with the tips of the fingers meeting in the middle. (It's fine to use just the pointer and the middle finger, but you may want to include the ring finger to make sure your forehead stays extra flat.)

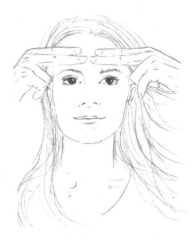

2. Use the strength of your fingers to place pressure against the forehead as you push your eyebrows up toward the hairline. Each time you raise and drop your eyebrows equals one forehead push-up (5 to 10 repetitions).

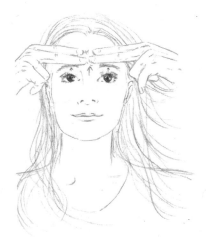

Cupping

To learn more about facial exercises and facial massage techniques, I recommend reading Tonya Zavasta's guide, *Rawsome Flex,* in which she describes massage techniques that strengthen the facial muscles and tissue quality.

Another great tool for strengthening and sculpting the facial structure is cupping massage. This ancient Chinese and Russian healing treatment increases the peripheral circulation of your blood, lymph, and interstitial fluid, improving metabolism and respiration of the skin. Cupping massage can be used on the face or the body, and is highly recommended for the treatment of cellulite problem areas. Just be sure to use only facial cups on the face. I like the Venus Body Sculpting Cups for the body and the Bellabaci cups for the face (see the Forever Beautiful Shopping Guide).

After oiling the skin well with argan or coconut oil, place the cup on the skin and create a light suction by squeezing the bulb. Gently run the suctioned cup up and down the cheek, thigh, calf, or other treatment area. Massage your chosen area for ten minutes at a light suction, working up to twenty minutes of heavier suction after the first several times.

Cupping may leave some bruising or reddish marks, so work gradually up to a longer treatment time and higher suction power. Bruising is an indication that the cupping is working; the weaker and more fatty the tissue, the more likely it is to respond with dark bruising. You'll feel and see the cupping working immediately. As the suction lifts the skin into the cup and makes the skin look "marbleized," it is pulling fresh blood into that skin. It feels intense and can even hurt in areas, but the pain should dissipate immediately upon moving the suction to another area, leaving the treated area feeling as if it's received a well-needed massage. After the first four weeks of continuous daily use, you should start to see cellulite gradually diminish. Many people notice cellulite diminishing much sooner than that. At any rate, consistency is key!

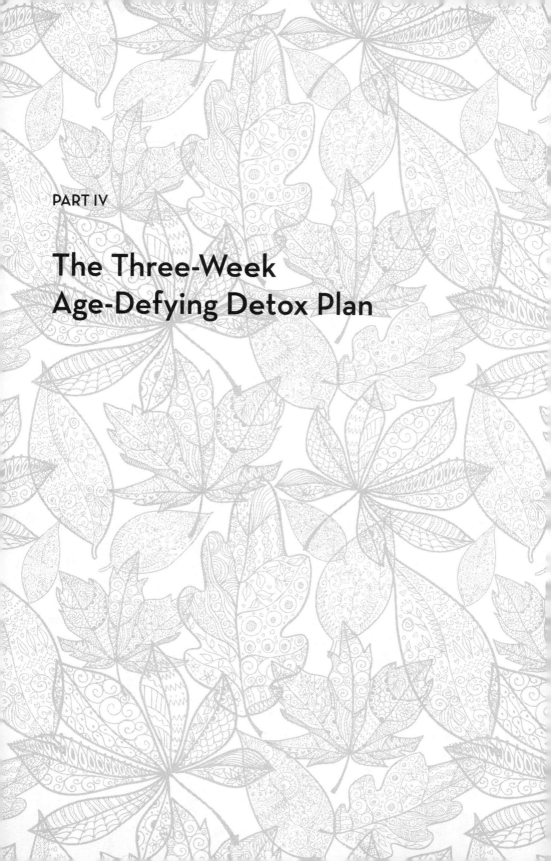

PART IV

The Three-Week
Age-Defying Detox Plan

Below you will find a three-week plan to help you establish new perceptions and habits. The plan is not an end in and of itself. Rather, it is designed as a guided initiation for those of you who wish to embark on a youth-regenerating path but aren't quite sure where to begin. Remember, the age-defying detox method is not about rigidity, dieting, or fitness. The intention is to ease you into a youth-regenerating lifestyle by letting the benefit of each reflection, meal, and activity really sink in and meld together. If you genuinely apply yourself to just three weeks of the method, you will experience a profound transformation that can set you on course for life.

For each week, I've laid out a sample day of activities followed by daily reflections and meal plans to serve as a blueprint for the whole seven days. This blueprint is followed by additional suggestions for you to draw from in order to tailor subsequent days to your personal preferences and needs.

While all three weeks will share elements of all five principles of timeless beauty, each one will have its own focus. During Week 1, we will place special emphasis on achieving clarity and adopting youth-regenerating values. During Week 2, we will shift our focus to increasing conductivity and life force in the body through movement and cellular cleansing. During Week 3, we will find fun and fulfilling ways to ritualize the various aspects of age-defying detox method in your daily schedule, extending them to include family and community, so that it takes firm root in your whole lifestyle.

By the end of the three weeks, you will have done some very deep transformative work on all levels of your being. If after you've completed the three-week plan you wish to repeat it to keep yourself on track, I highly recommend you do so. It will help to establish a rhythm and strengthen your commitment to this lifestyle. You will know when you're ready to guide yourself, much as you knew as a child when you were ready to ride your bike without training wheels, or when you could swim on your own. Remember how exhilarating that felt? Just imagine how amazing it will feel to gain your youth-regenerating wings!

Refer to the sample day of each week as often as necessary to keep the protocol alive in your mind over the entire three-week period, and just keep at it until you're flying high, implementing the practical applications and holding fast to the principles all on your own. Once you reach this point, please let us know via e-mail at Natalia@detoxtheworld.com, so our entire Detox the World team can celebrate with you!

But first, before we delve into the specific activities, reflections, and meal plans of the first week, here is an overview of the daily meal schedule you will be observing throughout the three weeks.

First Intake: After a night's sleep, rehydrate with a glass of pure water. Drink to quench your thirst. As you begin consuming more water-containing plant foods, your thirst will naturally decrease. However, you must have some pure water throughout the day, and water hydrates most effectively when your system is still and empty—i.e., before you consume anything else. You don't have to drink water as soon as you wake up if you're not thirsty. Just think of water as the first thing to take in when you feel the need for substance. Hydrate first and then enjoy the other wonderful drinks and foods in your day.

Morning Juice: Drink a tall glass of fresh, organic, raw vegetable juice. Try your favorite blend or mine, Green Lemonade (page 183).

Mid-morning Fruit or Juice (as desired): You may enjoy several pieces of fresh fruit if you are certain you do not have a problem with yeast (aka, candida) in your system. Otherwise, enjoy more vegetable juice if your body

---

Fruit and Yeast

If you want something more than juice during the morning but are concerned about a systemic yeast overload, choose lower-sugar fruits. (For further reading about a yeast-conscious approach, see my book Detox 4 Women.) Green apples, grapefruit, and berries are good low-sugar fruit options. Ripe bananas are also a great breakfast transition food; while they are not a low-sugar fruit per se, they are very filling, not aggressively cleansing like wet fruits, and, provided they are in fact ripe, they will have a gentle laxative effect on the bowel. (Note: Bananas are considered ripe when no longer green and covered with a dusting of brown freckles.) If you do include fruit in your daily diet, try to enjoy it sometime following your juice to maintain a light-to-heavy order of intake, and consume it alone on an empty stomach.

calls out for it in the morning hours. You may also enjoy herbal teas and/or lemon water as desired. Add NuNaturals stevia for sweetness rather than yeast-feeding sugars or syrups.

Light Midday Meal: Enjoy as much fresh, raw, organic vegetable salad as you like. The salad should be a base of organic leafy greens such as baby romaine or mesclun, topped with your favorite water-containing raw veggies, such as tomatoes, cucumbers, shredded carrots, sprouts, etc. To make it hearty, add one to two Hass avocados. You may also enjoy this salad with an oven-baked (not microwave-nuked) sweet potato and/or your favorite steamed vegetables.

Food-Combining Cheat Sheet

Starches include grains and starchy vegetables (potatoes, sweet potatoes, corn, squash, etc.). Starches combine with all raw and cooked vegetables and avocado.

Proteins include goat and sheep dairy, fish, eggs, and game meats. Proteins combine with all raw vegetables and all cooked non-starchy vegetables (eggplant, broccoli, kale, asparagus, etc.).

Legumes include lentils, peas, and beans. Legumes combine with all raw and cooked vegetables.

Dried fruits, nuts, and seeds include unsulfured organic dried fruits, raw seeds and seed butters (such as tahini, hemp, or sunflowerseed butter), raw nuts, and nut butters. (Note: Peanuts are technically part of the legume family, but we typically categorize them as nuts.) These foods combine with bananas and all raw vegetables. Dried fruits also combine with avocado (as in the case of a raw salad with raisins and avocado), but nuts and seeds do not.

Fruits combine only with other fruits and raw leafy greens. However, bananas and avocado can combine with starches or dried fruit.

Also consider the many different vegetable soups you could easily prepare to accompany your raw vegetable salad. Chop or puree your favorite cooked vegetables with vegetable stock and your favorite herbs and spices. For a little crunch, add some high-quality whole-grain crackers such as ak-mak, kale chips, or raw flax crackers. Do your best to adhere to good food-combining rules. Refer to the Food-Combining Cheat Sheet opposite for basic principles. (For further reading on this topic, refer to my previous books, *The Raw Food Detox Diet* or *Detox 4 Women*.)

Heavier Midday Meal Alternative: Should you desire something heavier for lunch, you could enjoy an organic whole-egg omelet. For best results, start with some raw leafy greens, such as a small version of the salad recommended above for the light midday meal, then use three to four eggs depending on your level of hunger. Be sure you are using only whole organic eggs, not any kind of egg substitute or just egg whites. You may use a pat of butter to cook them with, and you may enjoy your omelet with any low-starch vegetables.

Afternoon Pick-Me-Up (if needed): Sip your favorite herbal tea with stevia and/or a few squares of organic dark chocolate. Even better options would be a glass of pure, raw coconut water or another raw vegetable juice, or a raw blended smoothie or soup. Chopped raw vegetables (crudités), such as carrot and celery sticks, are also recommended.

Evening Meal: Enjoy a youth-regenerating dinner of your favorite raw and cooked vegetables with your favorite herbs and spices. Then, if desired, using the rules of good food combining, you may enjoy an animal protein (high-quality fish, organic eggs, or raw goat or sheep cheese) or a starch (baked yams, baked winter squash, or high-quality grains such as millet, quinoa, and buckwheat). Eat heartily until you are satiated, but take care not to overeat. I know, this may be easier said than done, but if you eat mindfully, and if you have released the negativity, discordance, and impurities from the day, you will find it much easier to do so.

Dessert: For dessert, enjoy one to two ounces of high-quality dark chocolate of at least 70 percent or more cocoa content. (My favorites are the Endangered Species brand or The Rose Bar, which we make by hand in small batches in a secluded beach village in South Africa using the best chocolate from all over the world!) Or, if you've had a raw-vegan meal, you can enjoy some raw nondairy ice cream made from coconut, banana, nut, or seed butters. For some raw dessert recipes, see page 211.

How Do You Know When You're Satiated?

If you have struggled with overeating or dietary restrictions, it may be hard to understand what true satiation feels like. You will know when you are full if you listen to your body without distraction. Here are some guiding tips:

Don't drink a lot of liquid while you eat. *In addition to diluting the digestive fluids in the stomach, drinking will create a false feeling of fullness that may leave you unsatisfied later.*

Take your time. *After finishing a moderately sized meal, take ten to twenty minutes to sit with it before you immediately go for seconds. Sometimes the brain doesn't register the meal right away, so let it catch up before you decide if you need more.*

Eat without stimulation. *Eating while driving, watching a movie, or having an emotional conversation engages your body and mind separately when they need to be working together. Take time out for your meals, so that work, entertainment, and stressful tasks don't interfere with mindful eating.*

Notice that all the midday meals are interchangeable with one another, as are all the evening meals. Just try not to swap midday meals for evening meals, since the former are more raw and water-containing whereas evening meals are generally more cooked and dense. This "light to heavy" pattern is designed for optimal digestion and energy.

Please also note that all meals are listed in order of intake rather than at given hours. This is because it's important to eat according to the body's call for sustenance, not by the clock. You'll notice that your natural tendencies will change as your body undergoes cellular regeneration. You'll see those old ingrained habits disappear as you release the density from your body and purge the addictive substances from your blood and tissues.

If you would like to lighten the diet further, and you feel fully prepared physically and emotionally to do so, you may enjoy midday meal suggestions in the evening as well. You might find that you'd rather skip an afternoon snack, or leave out the tea; that's fine, as long as you are listening to your body. However, the raw vegetable juices are nonnegotiable because they deliver the most powerful life force and alkaline hydration for the "awaken" part of the cleansing method.

Fish and Eggs

Fish and eggs have always had a place in the detox lifestyle for my clients who are transitioning away from mainstream fare. Including fish and eggs makes it easy to eat out and feel satiated, and it assuages the fears some people have about undertaking a mostly plant-based diet. However, it's important to note that truly clean, organic fish and eggs are not easily procured today. Our waters are polluted planet-wide, making even wild fish a questionable choice. "Free-range" eggs rarely means the hens are free to roam in wide-open organic pastures. They may be "uncaged" but crowded into coops with thousands of other chickens. Further, their feed, while organic, may still be made up of questionable ingredients. While I include fish and eggs in the recipe section and in this three-week plan to offer a range of options, I recommend cutting back gradually on flesh foods in general, until you are no longer dependent on them to feel satiated. Eventually, you'll find that salads, cooked vegetables, creamy tahini dressings, avocados, and the like will satisfy you and your cells much more in the long run!

WEEK 1: CLARITY

The theme of this first week is clarity. This is the time to start clearing away the clutter of your thoughts and your personal space to make way for the powerful insights and freedom of movement that you've been denying yourself for too long. Remember when you were very young and everything seemed fresh and new? Get ready to discover that feeling again! Embrace it. Some of this week's protocol may feel a bit strange to you, but an important part of rejuvenation is seeing yourself and the world with fresh eyes. Prioritize your morning reflections and let each one set the tone for the rest of the day. Ease into a gentle daily rhythm that allows you to experience the benefits of each exercise and take note of which ones resonate most with you. This week is all about self-discovery. Tune in to your body, to your surroundings, to the people you love. Start to clear away whatever is extraneous in your life (and in your pantry!) so you can open yourself up to what really matters.

Daily Activities for Week 1

Awaken: Awaken with praise and gratitude for the vessel of life force that you are! Let your first thought be the most inspirational one you can call to mind. It might be of the family that you love and nurture, or of the beautiful setting of your home, or of a creative passion that elevates your spirit. It might be a beloved friend or an admired historical figure, or perhaps an achievement that makes you feel proud and powerful. Find the inspiration that will fuel your desire to live fully. A passion for life is fundamental to timeless beauty. The greater your desire to live, the more life force will flood your veins; and the more life force, the more breakthroughs you will experience. Rise and shine, literally, and begin your day with presence, awareness, and self-sovereignty. Think of all that you will enjoy about the day.

Splash Your Face: Splash your face with cold water to clear away any cares or worries that may have kept you awake late or surfaced in your dreams, along with any negative energetic imprintings from the night. Do not underestimate the power of washing your face to clear away residual energies and start the day afresh. Clean ocean water is ideal, if you happen to live near the ocean, but cold tap water is fine for these purposes too.

Enjoy Five Minutes of Body Brushing: Body brushing with a natural-bristle body brush speeds up the process of cellular turnover, helps the dermal layers to shed old and dry skin cells, increases the flow of blood to the skin, and aids in the skin's detoxification process by stimulating lymphatic drainage. It is a powerful rejuvenating tool, and an invigorating way to start the day. Start with small brisk strokes on the bottoms of the feet and work your way up the legs, making long strokes up the calves and shins (like you're shaving your legs), followed by long strokes up the thighs in the same motion. Focus particular attention on the major lymph areas—the backs of the knees and the groin. Then address the arms, starting with lengthwise strokes on the palms. Work your way up each arm toward the heart center, paying special attention to the nodes under the armpit. Avoid the more-tender skin of the face and breasts, and use a gentle clockwise circular stroke on the stomach to mimic intestinal movement. In five minutes you've just given yourself a powerful lymphatic massage!

Empty Your Bowels: If you haven't already emptied your bowels, the body brushing (and inversions, which we will spotlight later on page 111) should help to stimulate them for elimination. If you do not eliminate significantly on your own, you may want to use this time to self-administer an enema or get a colonic.

Cleanliness

Most of us brush our teeth, wash our faces, and shower and shampoo once or twice a day. Yet most of this filth that we're washing away is coming from within. So why do we routinely ingest filthy substances that stress our filters—the skin, scalp, mouth, ears, nose, liver, kidneys, and bowels? Why do we only wash our outer surfaces? Most commercial ideas of cleanliness are illusions that can do more harm than good. We can brush and rinse our teeth with chemicals that promise the most extreme clean and scrub our skin with the most powerful soap and remain just as internally filthy as before. The fact is, we would do better to cake ourselves in pure mud than to scrub ourselves with harsh chemicals. Remember, cleanliness is an internal state, not just a cosmetic one.

Rebound and/or Exercise: Now that you are feeling open and clear, you may already feel like you're bouncing without the help of springs! However, now is the perfect time to do your exercise for the day, and certainly the best time to rebound if you have decided to make that part of your regular routine (which I highly recommend). Rebounding is uniquely beneficial for regeneration and detoxification because of the "squeeze" you feel at the bottom of a jump right before you bounce up, and at the top of the jump right before you come down. Each cell in the body is being wrung out, the lymphatic system massaged, and the digestive system stimulated. Additionally, because it is so low-impact, you get an intensive chi-generating workout without stressing the joints, bones, and organs.

Shower: Shower with pure soap made of all-natural plant-based ingredients. The alkalinity of pure soap picks up acidic by-products passed through the skin. This is a vital practice after working up a significant sweat, whether after rigorous exercise or time in the sauna. Your sweat is acidic and pure soap is alkaline, so the soap will magnetize the acidic waste up and off the skin. This is essential for ensuring that any toxins you've released in your sweat fully leave your body. If you're feeling up to it, try a cold shower right out of the sauna and then reward yourself after with a nice warm-hot finish

> ### Body Tip
> *Pay careful attention to what products you are using. Remember that chemicals can give you a false sense of cleanliness while breaking down your cell structure and speeding the aging process. I recommend a very simple body-cleansing protocol of body brushing and washing with pure soap and water. I find it especially invigorating to use scrubbing gloves to work the soap deeply into the skin to stimulate chi flow. Then I top myself off with coconut oil, cedar oil, or any other natural botanical oil that feels right; there are many excellent ones on the market. (For specific recommendations, see the Forever Beautiful Shopping Guide.) Clean oil feels wonderful on the skin and provides some aromatherapy to maximize well-being.*

(and then a final cold blast if you're really on a roll). I don't do this every time, but when I do I always feel tremendously euphoric in the hours that follow, as it stimulates even more chi flow!

Daily Re-centering: Exercise ways to maintain your center as you proceed through your day. Traditional meditation, recapitulation exercises, and delta- and theta-wave meditations (see page 61 and the Forever Beautiful Shopping Guide for recommendations) can be powerful re-centering tools. There are many to choose from, of varying lengths and methods, so experiment to see what works best with the energetic makeup of your mind and body.

If elements of your office life or other daytime environment conflict with your youth-regenerating ideals, recognize them as sources of friction that can enable you to grow, and then see if you can shift them into more-harmonious alignment. Rise gracefully to the challenge. The goal is to continually regenerate and evolve, not to chase a state of elusive perfection.

Life pulses with light and dark, alkalinity and acidity, input and output, degeneration and regeneration; the powerful interplay of yin and yang makes life dynamic and full of possibility. It requires great clarity to hold your flame and walk your truth in a place that challenges it, among people who run their energy in discordant, degenerating ways. It is a great challenge worthy of great self-possession. Accept the challenge and enjoy what you can learn from it. This week, your learning curve will be tremendous!

After-work/Pre-dinner Cleansing: Change out of your day clothes, and bathe or shower away any residues (the skin excretes toxins all day long), physical and energetic, that you've picked up from your daytime environments. Use pure soap or sea salts. You may follow with body brushing if you like. Re-harmonize any area of your being that may have been knocked off center over the course of the day.

If you have a home full of needs to be met, establish the ten, fifteen, or twenty minutes you need for this cleansing as an essential part of your evening ritual. Let others in your household know.

If you have young kids, teach them to help themselves to easily accessible fruit or vegetable snacks before you tend to their dinner. Give them as many age-appropriate tasks as you can to get those items off your to-do list. Remember to praise them for carrying out these tasks well and for easing

Energetic Imprintings
Energetic imprintings are areas of accumulated energy in the facial tissues—the eyes, the temples, the cheeks, and the lips—which hold the day's tensions. Energy must be fluid for it to be life-generating; stagnant energy is the harbinger of ills, both spiritual and cosmetic. Whatever tensions or imprintings you feel in your face at the end of the day or after a night's sleep indicate energetic obstructions. You can help to release them with gentle targeted facial massages in the evening (tracing circles around the areas where you feel the most pent-up energy and muscle tension), and clear them away with cold water in the morning.

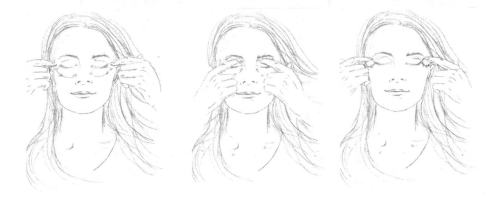

the burden on you. Children love being empowered to make a difference in their parents' lives.

Cleansing rituals are ubiquitous in nature—watch cats and birds do it! You, too, are entitled to taking moments out of your "hunting and gathering" schedule to reset your energies before moving into the evening's activities. If the stresses and toxic residues that we accumulate on a daily basis were visible to the naked eye, our culture would recognize them as the giant vampires they are. It would be considered basic hygienic practice to wash them away and rebalance the body at the end of each day.

Bath-Time Reflection

Take a moment to stand before the mirror and ask yourself, "Why am I here? What is it that I w]ant to change? What do youth and beauty mean to me?" Speak from the heart, even if it's painful.

How many of your self-judgments are fed by marketplace notions of youth and beauty? Do you perceive and treat yourself as an awkward assemblage of imperfect parts in desperate need of repair? Or do you perceive and treat yourself as a miraculous self-renewing organism deserving of respect and gratitude?

Then, as you bathe away the dirt and stress of the day, imagine dissolving away all the harsh judgments and points of negativity in your mind as well. As the tension in your muscles yields to the voluptuous heat of the water, as your skin tingles with its soothing entropy, consider how much joy you are capable of experiencing in your body when you treat it with respect and gentleness. Consider the ripples of positivity that could radiate from that if you let them.

Imagine having the clarity of mind to nurture yourself with respect, gentleness, and purity all the time, not just at bath time. What changes would that require? What would the implications be for your whole life experience? How would you see yourself differently?

Bedtime Ritual: As you prepare for bed, boost your skin's regenerating powers by cleansing your face (I recommend clearing makeup away with coconut butter followed by soap or cleanser) and then applying your favorite night serum for maximum overnight healing and hydration. Going to bed without cleansing and moisturizing your skin gives toxic residues the opportunity to work into your skin and cells while you sleep.

Be sure that your stomach is empty (or at least not full) when you go to bed so your body can take full advantage of the healing cycles that take place through the course of a full night's sleep. Ideally, if you want to honor your body's natural circadian rhythms, try to go to sleep by ten p.m., and remember to lie as flat and straight on your back as possible. Assuming some movement from side to side, sleeping flat ensures optimal circulation while you sleep. Also, gravity tugs enough on your face and neck during the day without you wedging your head up on thick pillows at night.

If you fall asleep the moment your head hits the pillow, that's a sign of over-exhaustion. Ideally, you will be able to fall asleep gradually. After you turn out the light, think beautiful thoughts or speak softly and kindly to your partner; you might express gratitude for something he/she did during the day that made you feel understood and appreciated. If you don't have a partner, focus on some act of kindness that you experienced during the day, or on something you've done that made you feel particularly good. You will soon drift off to sleep naturally.

If you are having trouble sleeping, or reaching deeper states of sleep, try shutting off all sources of artificial lighting as much as possible. If there is a lot of light seeping in from streetlights outside, draw the window curtains securely and make sure electronic devices are switched off or away from your bed. A good night's sleep is essential to youth regeneration, so create an environment that is conducive to it.

Daily Reflections for Week 1

Reflection upon rising, Day 1: Before you get out of bed, become fully present in your body. Do you feel rested and restored, or are you still carrying the physical burdens of yesterday? Remember your commitment to regenerating your body. Tell yourself: *I may do things today that I have never done before. I may live differently today than I normally do. I may reflect on concepts today that I have not entertained seriously before. These activities and experiences will all be for my highest good, and I'm excited to start this adventure!*

Reflection upon rising, Day 2: Note how you feel this morning compared to yesterday. Try to feel your cells ringing with life. Can you feel the subtle vibratory hum? That hum is available to you anytime you wish to tune in to it. It can rebalance you in seconds. Send your cells a wave of appreciation that they can feel. Generate as much love as you can for them. Feel them ring back to you. Note that you are fully able to communicate with them. Know that your choices today will bring them into greater harmony and increased power.

Reflection upon rising, Day 3: You may have heard the saying, "Energy flows where attention goes." Keeping this in mind, consider that you are the gardener of your own personal garden and you are caring for your soil, roots, shoots, and blossoms. What are you sowing and reaping? If you stock up on needless fertilizers, pesticides, and fancy equipment, you'll reap debt and clutter, guilt and toxicity. If you till the soil, water your plants with pure goodness, and give them enough room to breathe in the sunlight, you will reap classic, radiant beauty. The age-defying detox method is a more evolved, enlightened way of gardening. It brings you back to your roots as a radiant creature who drinks in the sun's energy. Today, how will you continue to sow the seeds of health, beauty, and buoyancy?

Reflection upon rising, Day 4: Before you get out of bed, take a minute to think about everyone in your life for whom you feel unconditional love. Think of how much joy and nourishment each one brings to your life. No matter what any of them might have done to disappoint you in the past, let your heart swell with love and forgiveness for them. Doesn't it feel good? Now, can you feel that same unconditional love for yourself? Or are you holding on to stories about yourself, about your family, about your cultural identity that tell you who and what and how you are—or should be? How many negative labels have you collected along the way? From this day forward, you will work to dissolve them with each thought and action. There is no place here for labels, blame, judgment, or deflating stories. The path of rejuvenation is one of self-love and self-liberation. How far down that path will you travel today?

Reflection upon rising, Day 5: Today, commit yourself to practicing compassion. Start before you get out of bed by promising to be compassionate to yourself. Recognize some of the cruel names you call yourself in your darker moments and take an honest look at the standards you hold yourself to. Would you ever call someone you loved those names, or hold him or her to the same standards of perfection? Take a moment to reflect on this, and then forgive yourself. Set aside judgment for the day, and be gentle and understanding with your limitations and actions. Carry this same spirit of compassion into all of your interactions with others today.

Reflection upon rising, Day 6: Use this time to think about your body strictly in terms of utility. Today, instead of dwelling on the superficial or cosmetic aspects of your body, you will focus on all that it can do. What parts of you are the strongest? Can you rely on your sturdy legs to get where you need to go? Are your hands adept at creating things? Do you have admirable stamina for playing with your children? Review the day ahead with gratitude for all of the ways that your physical self supports the life you've chosen.

Reflection upon rising, Day 7: Recap your week of morning reflections. What have you done this week that you've never done before? As a result, do you feel your cells ringing with more vibrancy? Do you feel that you are "tilling the soil" to let in more nutrients? Do you feel yourself opening up to greater love and compassion? Are you growing in appreciation for your body? In light of all this, today you will be very mindful of the language you use, trading in those old negative labels for words of inspiration. Picture the sun's energy coursing through your cells, and remember all of the strength and support your body gives you. Commit to not using negative words when referring to yourself, in speech or in thought. Your vocabulary will be loving, compassionate, and kind.

Daily Menus for Week 1

This week ride the wave of inspiration by trying out new foods and recipes. You can begin with the recipes in this book (see page 179). Explore your local health-food store, and trade up to higher-quality whole foods and pantry items that will complement your daily menus. Try your hand at raw desserts, and challenge your palate to find the pleasure in simplicity. You can of course follow these sample menus to the letter if this makes your life easier, but by all means feel free to experiment and swap out any items as you see fit to keep your taste buds happy!

DAY 1

Juice Time: Natalia's Classic Green Lemonade

Optional: Mid-morning fruit

Midday Meal: Natalia's Favorite Raw Salad, followed by a bowl of Vegetable Soup Perfection

Afternoon Pick-me-up: Juice, crudités (e.g., raw celery or carrot sticks), a cabbage or romaine leaf wrap-up, or herbal tea

Evening Meal: Classic Avocado Salad, followed by Sweet Butternut Heaven

Dessert: Raw Chocolate Pudding

Crudités

Raw vegetables are the ideal afternoon snack. Make yourself a crudités platter of your favorite chopped raw vegetables for a delicious mini meal. Some great options are celery sticks, carrot sticks, peeled and sliced beets or yams, red, yellow, or orange bell peppers, jicama, and cucumber. You can add some sliced raw goat cheddar or homemade avocado guacamole if you need something more substantial.

DAY 2

Juice Time: The Great Eliminator

Optional: Mid-morning fruit

Midday Meal: Avocado Soup and Salad, optionally with ak-mak crackers, or followed by one to two bananas

Afternoon Pick-me-up: Crudités with or without
Simple Raw Guacamole

Evening Meal: Tahini Delight

Dessert: Raw Vanilla Ice Cream

DAY 3

Juice Time: The Great Rejuvenator

Optional: Mid-morning fruit

Midday Meal: Ginger Ivory Splendor Soup, followed by Chlorophyll-Banana Milk Shake

Afternoon Pick-me-up: Raw jewel or garnet yam, peeled and sliced and eaten either plain or with raw tahini dressing/dip (from Tahini Delight salad recipe)

Evening Meal: Tender Baby Salad with avocado, followed by half of a baked butternut squash

Dessert: Pumpkin Pie in a Bowl

DAY 4

Juice Time: Clean Bloody Mary

Optional: Mid-morning fruit

Midday Meal: Raw Roma and Basil Soup with optional ak-mak crackers or Sweet Potato Toast

Afternoon Pick-me-up: Carob-Spinach-Banana Shake

Evening Meal: Mexican Salad, followed by Eggplant Pizzas served with steamed baby spinach

Dessert: One generous scoop of Laloo's goat's milk ice cream

DAY 5

Juice Time: Good Morning Mojito

Optional: Mid-morning fruit

Midday Meal: Crystal-Filled Key Lime Pie, followed by Green Log in the Sun

Afternoon Pick-me-up: Raw jewel or garnet yam, peeled and sliced and eaten either plain or with raw tahini dressing/dip; or Carob-Spinach-Banana Shake

Evening Meal: Harvest Salad followed by Simple Pasta Puttanesca

Dessert: Raw Strawberry Sorbet

DAY 6

Juice Time: Natalia's Classic Green Lemonade

Optional: Mid-morning fruit

Midday Meal: Creamy Avo-Ranch Salad, followed by Berry Young

Afternoon Pick-me-up: Juice, raw veggie crudités, a cabbage or romaine leaf wrap-up, or herbal tea

Evening Meal: Mediterranean Beet Salad followed by Garlic "Bread" Goat Melts

Dessert: Cheat Tiramisu

DAY 7

Juice Time: The Great Eliminator

Optional: Mid-morning fruit

Midday Meal: Tender Baby Salad, followed by Green Piña Colada

Afternoon Pick-me-up: Juice or crudités with Simple Raw Guacamole

Evening Meal: Natalia's Favorite Raw Salad, followed by the Color Melt

Dessert: Detox Minty Hot Chocolate

WEEK 2: CONDUCTIVITY AND LIFE FORCE

After a week on the youth-regenerating plan, you should be ready to ramp up your internal conductivity and life force. One of the most effective ways to do this is to release waste with the help of colonics and/or enemas. This may or may not appeal to you, but if you feel ready to take yourself to the next level of cellular regeneration by releasing all the waste you've awakened in the large intestine, this is a good time to go for it. If you don't have a bowel movement on your own for one to three days following a colonic, do not be concerned. This is very typical. Your bowel, which is not used to moving so much out at once, feels it can take a short vacation. As the accumulated waste is removed, it will get its mojo back! Remember, the bowel is a huge muscle, and when it flexes to carry waste through, it is called peristalsis. The bowel can be unpredictable as it makes this transition from sluggish to strong and healthy. Your job is to make sure that all the garbage keeps moving out. This is the single most effective way to increase conductivity and clear the way for abundant life force.

Daily Activities for Week 2

The following activities may take the place of the activities introduced in Week 1. However, you are welcome and encouraged to continue the previous week's exercises alongside the following ones as you feel comfortable doing so.

Visualize: Light outside. Light inside. Light all around you. Light within you. Feel your skeletal system as the powerful superconductor it is. Imagine filling your marrow with electromagnetic chi. Enjoy the warm, tingling sensation. Imagine the light emitting from your bones through your skin like the sun's rays, from your whole body. Like the sun, you emit great currents of energy, warmth, and light. Your singular shining life is worth infinitely more than all of society's petty stressors put together. You have the power to overcome those stressors, but first you must see them for what they are: illusions. Make a pact with yourself that from now on you will operate from your radiant center, not from the directives imposed upon you by cultural norms. You will exercise your power to choose your own thoughts, actions, communications, and experiences; others will not choose them for you. You will remain present with your inner light and let it shine powerfully on all that comprises your life.

Sauna: After "taking out the garbage" through the colon, maximizing chi flow with your favorite whole-body exercise, and supporting lymph release through rebounding and body brushing, your body is open and ready to expel any remaining residues through the skin via a deep sweat. If you have, or have access to, an infrared sauna, sweating out toxins in a sauna is the perfect next activity. Traditional saunas (typically found at gyms and spas) are also wonderful, but they don't produce the same deep detox as a far-infrared sauna, which heats the core of the body to stimulate the expulsion of toxins at the deepest level. Thirty minutes to an hour is the ideal amount of time to get the benefits of a sauna, but if you're a beginner, start with only fifteen to twenty minutes, and build from there as your comfort level allows. Do not exceed one hour.

Shower: Showering is essential after a deep sweat, whether after some rigorous exercise or time in the sauna. Your acidic sweat will be purged through the skin and then magnetized by the alkalinity of pure soap. This will ensure that toxins released through the dermal layers fully leave your body. Then follow with a cold water blast to shrink the cells and shock the surface of the skin, releasing a last squeeze of trapped toxicity and sending blood and oxygen rushing through the body.

Centering before Dinner: During the first week, I asked you to remove your clothes and slip into a warm bath or shower to cleanse away the residues of the day and rebalance your energy. I did this for two reasons: 1) because you pull in much filth from modern living and excrete toxins through your skin over the course of the day; and 2) because your energetic aura is continually affected by what you pick up from other people, radiation, pollution, offices, schools, public centers, and commercial spaces. Now you can see how this ritual is essential to daily regeneration. Removing this residue is

Body Tip

The ears, jaw, hands, and feet are four areas that store up loads of the day's stresses and tensions. Just a few moments of massaging just one or all of these areas will shed much of the stagnant energy.

For the ears: *Place a thumb on the back of each ear, bending the pointer finger just inside the curve of the ear. Squeeze the thumb and pointer finger together against the ear in a rolling motion. You'll feel the trapped, stagnant energy release immediately.*

For the jaw: *Open your mouth as wide as you can, dropping your jaw straight down. As you open wide, you'll feel the negative energy release. Repeat three times, and do so again and again throughout the day as needed.*

For the hands: *Press the thumb of one hand into the palm of the opposite hand, with the four fingers pressing against the back of the hand. Massage the entire hand by moving the thumb to each point of the palm and fingers.*

For the feet: *The ideal time to do this is in the bath at the end of the day. Place your thumbs on the soles of your feet, wrapping your fingers around the tops of your feet, and squeeze until you've covered every point on your feet. If you are not in water, you may want to use some oil. But if you have nothing on hand, it is still heavenly and rebalancing!*

key to ensuring that you bring goodness to your evening, enjoy the people in your home, and savor a beautiful meal without overeating.

Clean Your Closet: Just as your body's pathways need to be cleared to conduct energy freely, your living space must also be cleared of needless and counterproductive items so you can inhabit it with joy and clarity. This is especially true of your clothes closet. What can you remove (i.e., throw away, give away, or sell) that is impeding the flow of your life? Take time to go through shelves and racks, asking yourself of each item: *Do I truly love this? Do I wear it? Does it make me feel good about myself? Does it reflect who I am becoming?* If you answer no to any of these questions, send it to the removal pile! If it's too tight or constrictive, uncomfortable, unflattering, or stress-inducing in any way, get rid of it. If you are serious about timeless beauty, there is no room in your closet for "skinny" clothing that doesn't fit, uncomfortable synthetic fabrics that don't let the skin breathe, or anything that makes you feel less than your best self. Once you've cleared the clutter, you will love stepping into your closet and picking out your clothes for the day!

Daily Reflections for Week 2

Reflection upon rising, Day 8: As you awake, consider your body's regenerative shifts and transformations during the night. What essential physical and mental functions do the hours of restful sleep in the quiet darkness facilitate and support? How do they differ from yet inform your physical and mental functions during the daylight hours? Take a moment to appreciate the fact that, day and night, your energies are deeply intertwined with your natural circadian rhythms. Given a chance, your body will respond beautifully and reliably to these rhythms of regeneration.

Reflection upon rising, Day 9: What youth-regenerating values will you consciously embrace today? Pick two or three that are especially important to you as you move further into your second week. In embracing these values, what values must you work to leave behind? Speak your intentions aloud. Some of the old self-destructive values may still have their hooks in you, which you'll know if you feel a catch in your breath or a flutter of anxiety in your stomach as you say them aloud. Why might this be? Follow the feeling to its origin. For example, you may say to yourself, "I value my self-sovereignty" and "I no longer depend on the judgments of others." If that latter statement rings false, you are probably still spinning your wheels trying to measure up. Take heart, for this means you've identified an obstruction. As you work to release the fear of judgment and supplant old degenerating values with youth-regenerating ones, you will experience a palpable uplift.

Reflection upon rising, Day 10: As you awake, consider your mental state. Do you feel rested and ready to leap into your day, or are you still tired and burdened with residual anxieties from yesterday? Why do you suppose that is? Remember how it felt as a young child to awaken completely refreshed, wide-eyed, and excited about the day ahead? Isn't it time you experienced that effortless buoyancy and optimism again? The problem is that inharmonious thoughts and feelings stick in the psyche just as dense, acidic foods stick in the cells and tissues. Thoughts are very much alive and energetically charged, even though you cannot see them. Whatever thoughts you feed will grow, take root, and send ripples throughout your whole life experience. Positive thoughts infuse you with energy and light, whereas negative thoughts can grow like parasites, obstructing clarity and kindness. Today, what will you do to starve the negative thoughts and feed your positive ones, so that you can awake tomorrow, and the next day, and the next, with childlike optimism?

Reflection upon rising, Day 11: Commit to spending today day focused on the most basic conductor of all: breathing. Pulling fresh oxygen into your lungs begins a series of events in the body that is truly awe-inspiring. This oxygen is essential to everything—from brain function to cleansing to healing. Then, when you exhale, your powerful lungs force the expulsion of carbon dioxide and begin to loosen old toxicity, including mucoid buildup, and even tarry buildup from cigarettes and car exhaust. Before you get out of bed, lie with your eyes closed and take ten deep breaths in a row, holding the air in at the end of the inhalation while focusing on an optimistic thought, and feeling the lungs fully empty at the bottom of the exhalation as they expel negativity. Now plan two other breaks in your day where you can take five to ten deep, cleansing breaths.

Reflection upon rising, Day 12: Focus today on extending your powers of conductivity to those around you. Can you send ripples of positive energy from your core to your family and friends . . . to your coworkers . . . to your larger community? How might you go about that? Plan a surprise for a loved one, tip a little extra, practice patient kindness in every interaction, or lend an ear to someone who needs it. Set your intention before you get out of bed, and decide to see how powerfully you can conduct genuine love to others today.

Reflection upon rising, Day 13: With your eyes closed, tap into the power of universal conductivity through a simple meditation. Feel the heat of the Earth's center warming you from below. Picture the soil that grows your food and the trees that give you oxygen. Draw a deep breath and let it out into the atmosphere. You are energetically linked to the whole world around you. Feel your cells vibrate with solar energy, absorbed through the skin and the plants you eat, fed with rain and soil. New energy is constantly being generated, and it flows through you and every living thing. This second week of cleansing is linking you more consciously back into this cycle, which is affording you the life force to regenerate. Feel this greater conductivity at work as you move through your day.

Reflection upon rising, Day 14: On this last day of your second week, bring your thoughts back to the minutiae of life. Look deep within your inner space, down to the subatomic level. Remember what you are doing: opening blocked pathways and restoring conductivity to every single atom, cell, organ, and system of the body. The root of joy starts with these tiniest sparks, which harmonize into a current, moving faster and stronger as conductivity increases and obstructions are cleared away. Create a clear mental picture of this joyful current of pure life force moving through your body. When you have moments of mental obstruction or self-doubt, come back to this picture to refresh and reaffirm the importance of what you are doing.

Daily Menus for Week 2

This week, begin to lighten your midday meals wherever it feels good to do so. Start to home in on what your favorite textures and flavors are. Pick out your three favorite recipes for each meal—recipes you could rotate into your schedule indefinitely that you know will leave you satisfied. Make these your go-to recipes on the days when you don't want to be creative or adventurous or think too much. Gradually, you'll develop new favorites and a sense of ease and fluency about eating for conductivity, but it's important to have reliable staples at any given time—especially during this initial three-week period—to help keep you on the youth-regenerating path.

DAY 8

Juice Time: Natalia's Classic Green Lemonade

Optional: Mid-morning fruit

Midday Meal: Harvest Salad, followed by Sunshine Joy

Afternoon Pick-me-up: Juice, crudités, a cabbage or romaine leaf wrap-up, or herbal tea

Evening Meal: Mediterranean Beet Salad, followed by Garlic "Bread" Goat Melts

Dessert: Cheat Tiramisu

DAY 9

Juice Time: Clean Bloody Mary

Optional: Mid-morning fruit

Midday Meal: Tahini Delight, followed by Raw Strawberry Sorbet

Afternoon Pick-me-up: Juice, crudités, a cabbage or romaine leaf wrap-up, or herbal tea

Evening Meal: Natalia's Favorite Raw Salad, followed by Eggplant Pizzas

Dessert: Detox Minty Hot Chocolate

DAY 10

Juice Time: The Great Rejuvenator

Optional: Mid-morning fruit

Midday Meal: Tender Baby Salad with avocado, followed by Raw Chocolate Pudding

Afternoon Pick-me-up: Juice, crudités, a cabbage or romaine leaf wrap-up, or herbal tea

Evening Meal: Mexican Salad, followed by Quickest Spaghetti

Dessert: One generous scoop of Laloo's goat's milk ice cream

DAY 11

Juice Time: Clean Bloody Mary

Optional: Mid-morning fruit

Midday Meal: Classic Avocado Salad, followed by Curry Corn Soup

Afternoon Pick-me-up: Juice, crudités, a cabbage or romaine leaf wrap-up, or herbal tea

Evening Meal: Natalia's Favorite Raw Salad, followed by a Western Omelet

Dessert: Two to four ounces of 70 percent dark chocolate

DAY 12

Juice Time: Good Morning Mojito

Optional: Mid-morning fruit

Midday Meal: Tahini Delight, followed by Grain-Free Asian Kombu Noodle Soup

Afternoon Pick-me-up: Juice, crudités, a cabbage or romaine leaf wrap-up, or herbal tea

Evening Meal: Detox Maple-Glazed Salmon served on a large bed of baby spinach with lemon juice, and a side of "water sautéed" broccoli

Dessert: One generous scoop of Laloo's goat's milk ice cream

Water Sautéing

Instead of sautéing vegetables in cooked oil, just use half an inch of water in the bottom of a lidded pan. Bring the water to a boil, add the vegetables, and cover. They will only need to be cooked three to five minutes to obtain a bright, vibrant color and a slightly soft, steamed consistency.

DAY 13

Juice Time: The Refresher

Optional: Mid-morning fruit

Midday Meal: Mexican Salad, followed by Raw Goat Cheese Sandwich

Afternoon Pick-me-up: Juice, crudités, or herbal tea

Evening Meal: Classic Avocado Salad, followed by Creamy Parsnip Soup

Dessert: Two to four ounces of 70 percent dark chocolate

DAY 14

Juice Time: Natalia's Classic Green Lemonade

Optional: Mid-morning fruit

Midday Meal: Ginger Ivory Splendor Soup, followed by a banana

Afternoon Pick-me-up: Juice, crudités, a cabbage or romaine leaf wrap-up, or herbal tea

Evening Meal: Mama Mia Pizza Salad, followed by Eggplant Pizzas

Dessert: Detox Minty Hot Chocolate

WEEK 3: LEVITY AND RITUAL

By this time, you're probably feeling noticeably lighter and freer in your body. Even if you are still craving certain acidic substances, your palate is cleaner, your mind is clearer, and your pathways are conducting more life force than they have in a long while—perhaps since you were a child! This week is the time to ramp up your game a notch by continuing everything that has been working for you in the past two weeks, but placing more focus on levity. Specifically, inversions and facial exercises will help to counteract the many hours each day that gravity is pulling down on your organs and facial features. They will improve circulation and help to tone areas of your body that you rarely think about. This is also the time to focus on ritualizing the principles and practices of timeless beauty. Find ways to integrate them seamlessly into your daily life, so that they will carry you comfortably well beyond this three-week initiation period into ever greater states of youthfulness and vitality.

Daily Activities for Week 3

Please continue with any of the daily activities that you love from the previous weeks. Make them a daily practice, alternating or swapping certain ones out as desirable or necessary. See if you can work your way up to incorporating all of them at least a few times a week. The trick is to find the sweet spot where your daily youth-regenerating exercises keep your body humming like a finely tuned instrument—neither overstressed nor collecting dust in the corner!

Practice an Inversion: Using a slant board or an inversion board, stretch your body out in an inverted position, with your feet 45 degrees above your shoulders, keeping your spine straight and aligned with the rest of your body. Notice how your perspective shifts and troubles dissolve when you're inverted. Feel the sensation of blood flowing to your heart and brain. Imagine the increased circulation throughout your whole body—how it stimulates hair growth, energizes your brain, releases tension, revitalizes your facial tissues, supports your lymphatic system to propel waste out of your cells and organs, and enables your cecum (in the lower right side of your colon) to release matter for quicker elimination. Take five to ten minutes (or as much time as you need) to feel the full gravity-defying benefits of this position.

Inversions should be done on a completely empty stomach, so enjoy them early in the morning, after a colonic, or at least four hours after a properly combined meal. Keep in mind that morning inversions help to set your perspective for the day ahead, and evening inversions can reduce stress and provide a reflective time to reset your energies after a long day.

Practice Facial Exercises: You can practice facial exercises (page 77) while you are doing just about anything, but unless you commit to a time to do them, chances are you won't. They are really easy to forget! I recommend making a point of doing them while bathing or practicing inversions.

Practice Mental Levity: Bring levity to your mind and heart by engaging only the most uplifting thoughts. Positive thinking has the power to open you up to love, gratitude, connectedness, vitality, and creativity. Indulging negative, gravity-laden thoughts, on the other hand, will only lead to disappointment, resentment, pessimism, and obstruction—weighing you down in both body and spirit. Remember to counteract the tug of gravity with mental levity.

Daily Reflections for Week 3

Reflection upon rising, Day 15: Consider how rejuvenation is in many ways synonymous with purification, but not in a neurotic, germaphobic way! As you stretch your body upon rising, hold the thought of purity in your mind as it pertains to every cell in your body and every thought in your mind. Call to mind the cleansing properties of warm sunlight, fresh mineral springs, cool alkaline air, and how your body intuitively responds to these things. The problem is that we live in a world fraught with man-made toxicity, and as long as that's the case, the key to timeless beauty is to neutralize the impurities of our daily lives through restorative cleansing rituals. Instead of feeling exasperated and sorry for yourself to be living in such a toxic age, let your heart swell with gratitude that you are now well fortified with the knowledge and tools of purification!

Reflection upon rising, Day 16: Start today with a very simple gratitude list. While you can certainly reflect on this in your mind, it will be a much more meaningful exercise to write the gratitude list down. What are your greatest blessings and joys? Do you have a wonderful home, loving family, caring friends, or affectionate animal companions? Are there certain aspects of your life that make you feel lucky and fulfilled? List it all, great and small, in no particular order. You can feel grateful for something as silly as your favorite pair of jeans or as profound as the interconnectedness of all living things. Keep it concise and simple. You can practice this reflection at various points throughout the day—while waiting in line at a store, for example, or during moments of stress or emotional pain. Let your feelings of gratitude this morning radiate throughout the rest of your day.

Reflection upon rising, Day 17: Start today by visualizing the day ahead with optimism and a determination to succeed, but also with a promise of gentleness toward your limitations. Run through your day in your mind, one task at a time. Picture your beautiful and serene morning, your delicious meals, your interactions with others. See yourself shining at work or in conversation with friends and family, and responding with love to challenging moments. Just as a professional runner will run a course in his or her mind before a race, you can walk yourself mentally through your own course. Picture all the important steps that will lead you to a wonderful sense of personal fulfillment this evening.

Reflection upon rising, Day 18: Now that you have aligned your lifestyle with the principles of timeless beauty for many days, you can now start to pick and choose and prioritize the practical applications that work best for you. Reflect today on which reflections, exercises, and meals are sacred to you, and how you can cherish them. Remember, your priorities can and will likely change over time. For example, you may find yourself committed to your sauna and certain favorite meditations during the colder months, while you prefer daily rebounding and body brushing during other months. Before you get out of bed, decide which practices will be nonnegotiable today, and for the rest of the week. You can make changes and amendments as you progress, but commit to finding a way to honor these top priorities.

Reflection upon rising, Day 19: Start today by recalling what your original goals were when you first picked up this book. Were you feeling dissatisfied with your appearance? Was your body in pain, or feeling slow and weak? Were you feeling anxious about getting older? Remember why you embarked on this age-defying plan, and what hopes you brought with you. Are they the same goals you have today? Have any of them shifted or expanded at all? Right now, before you get out of bed, see if you can open yourself up to new goals that you may have discovered during this process. Now, in light of these future goals, set your present goals for today.

Reflection upon rising, Day 20: Focus this morning on your physical, spiritual, and emotional alignment. Our society's commerce functions by pulling these elements apart, treating the body as separate from the spiritual and emotional self, and even breaking those down into further parts. Spend ten minutes putting them back together through a body survey. Start with your feet: How do they feel? Are they hot or cold? Can you feel blood circulating in your feet? If your feet had emotions, what would they be? Feel their physicality through sensation, but also be receptive to any messages they may be sending to you: Do you sense frustration, or contentment, or perhaps an energetic impulse? Scan the entire body, moving up through the legs, to the thighs, and to the pelvis and abdomen. Then start at the fingertips and move inward until you reach the solar plexus. Lastly, start at the top of the head and scan over the face, through the neck, and down to the chest. Take as little or as much time as you need to begin your day with the lines of communication between all aspects of yourself open and connected. Make this body survey a weekly ritual.

Reflection upon rising, Day 21: Edgar Cayce was a healer who professed to be able to channel spirit voices. He diagnosed and treated thousands of serious illnesses and gave psychic readings to over nine thousand patients. But he always maintained that the best way to find answers was to get them from within. Reconnect with your innermost self today. Are there issues you've needed help with, questions you have, or decisions you're trying to make? You hold within you a deep source of wisdom and insight, and you alone can access it. Close your eyes and connect with your breath, and then connect with your core self, who has the highest good in mind for you. Shine a light on the issues you've been grappling with, and examine them from this perspective. You have the answers you need, even if the answer is sometimes to ask for outside help. Carry this conscious connection to your wise innermost self throughout the day.

Body Tip

Today, our skin is overexposed to intense weather, chemicals, stress, and radiation. The result: prematurely dry, exhausted skin. Keeping a coat of pure natural oil on clean skin protects it from this onslaught. If you are going out, you can remedy an oily sheen with a few pats of a cotton cloth. If you're in the privacy of your home, use the opportunity to apply a high-quality oil liberally after cleansing, and do so again after washing your face before bedtime. I have found this practice to be very effective in preventing wrinkles. If you are maintaining your internal health through diet and regular cleansing and using only the purest oils (e.g., virgin raw coconut oil, pure vitamin E oil, argan oil, and cedar oil from the Ringing Cedars of Russia), you will not likely break out. I use these oils day and night to keep my skin from drying out, especially during New York City winters—and I suffer neither breakouts nor wrinkles!

Daily Menus for Week 3

This week begin to think beyond your own meal plans by accommodating family members or friends and dining out. Share a favorite raw recipe with an appreciative friend, or see what happens if you switch your children's pasta to spelt or quinoa pasta. Look up the menus for favorite restaurants and practice building properly combined, clean, raw, or mostly raw meals from their options. This is a time to try being social with your new lifestyle, and introducing loved ones to the values and principles that are important to you. How can you make long-lasting changes by integrating the age-defying detox method into your home life, work life, and social life? This week is the time to look toward the future and hone your strategies for making personal regeneration a daily priority.

DAY 15

Juice Time: Natalia's Classic Green Lemonade

Midday Meal: Harvest Salad, followed by Berry Young

Afternoon Pick-me-up: Juice or herbal tea

Evening Meal: Mama Mia Pizza Salad, followed by
Ana's Favorite Frittata

Dessert: One generous scoop of Laloo's goat's milk ice cream

DAY 16

Juice Time: The Great Eliminator

Midday Meal: Avocado Soup and Salad, with Sweet Potato Toast

Afternoon Pick-me-up: Juice or herbal tea

Evening Meal: Mediterranean Beet Salad, followed by
Scallop Consommé

Dessert: Stevia-sweetened tea and two to four ounces of 70 percent dark chocolate

DAY 17

Juice Time: The Great Rejuvenator

Midday Meal: Harvest Salad, followed by Chlorophyll Banana Milk Shake

Afternoon Pick-me-up: Juice or herbal tea

Evening Meal: Tender Baby Salad with avocado, followed by Comforting Carrot and Sweet Potato Soup

Dessert: Raw Chocolate Pudding

DAY 18

Juice Time: Clean Bloody Mary

Midday Meal: Simple Pasta Puttanesca, followed by Crystal-Filled Key Lime Pie

Afternoon Pick-me-up: Juice or herbal tea

Evening Meal: Natalia's Favorite Raw Salad, followed by Simple Spiked Snapper

Dessert: Sliced raw goat cheddar cheese plate and two to four ounces of 70 percent dark chocolate

DAY 19

Juice Time: Good Morning Mojito

Midday Meal: Ginger Ivory Splendor Soup, followed by Green Log in the Sun

Afternoon Pick-me-up: Juice or herbal tea

Evening Meal: Mama Mia Pizza Salad, followed by Eggplant Pizzas

Dessert: Cheat Tiramisu

DAY 20

Juice Time: The Refresher

Midday Meal: Tender Baby Salad, followed by Pumpkin Pie in a Bowl

Afternoon Pick-me-up: Juice or herbal tea

Evening Meal: Creamy Avo-Ranch Salad, followed by two baked sweet potatoes with butter and sea salt

Dessert: Detox Minty Hot Chocolate

DAY 21

Juice Time: Natalia's Classic Green Lemonade

Midday Meal: Raw Roma and Basil Soup with
Raw Goat Cheese Sandwich

Afternoon Pick-me-up: Juice or herbal tea

Evening Meal: Classic Avocado Salad with Nama Shoyu soy sauce, followed by Spicy Curry

Dessert: Raw Chocolate Pudding

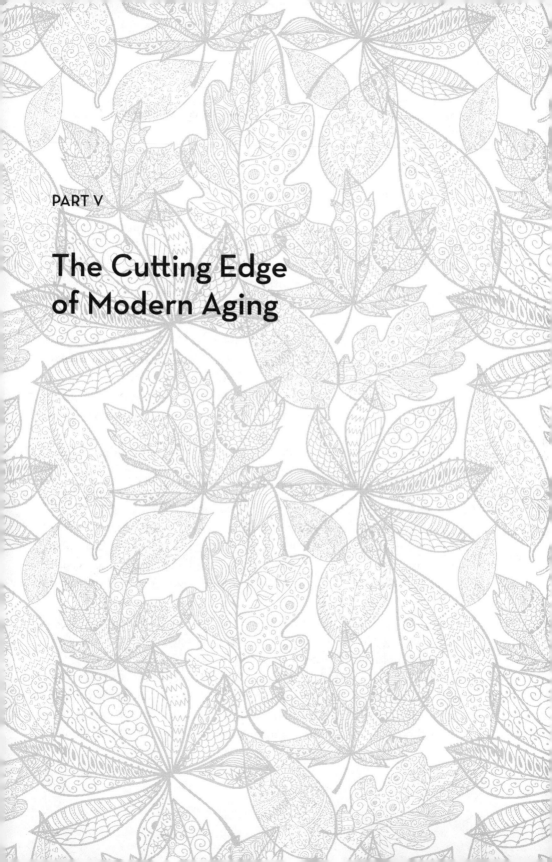

PART V

The Cutting Edge
of Modern Aging

Beyond mere cosmetic concerns, there are countless health concerns that are typically associated with aging. In our culture, to grow older is practically synonymous with making more doctors' visits, collecting more drug prescriptions, and becoming more susceptible to illnesses. The problem is that many of the drugs being prescribed today, while targeting one specific symptom, end up triggering other imbalances and further toxic accumulation. What modern medical practitioners tends to overlook is that the underlying cause of most disease in the body is obstruction: cells, tissues, organs, and pathways clogged with waste and by-products.

The modern lifestyle overexposes us to unfit foods, pharmaceuticals, and all manner of environmental chemicals, radiation, and pathogens that our bodies must constantly struggle to process. Any substance that enters the body that cannot be easily digested, assimilated, excreted, exhaled, or released through perspiration leaves behind a residue. The lymphatic system becomes overwhelmed, the skin appears blotchy and tired, and the intestine fills with impacted waste. This accumulation in the intestine causes indigestion, interferes with the growth of beneficial intestinal flora, and blocks nutrient absorption.

As long as our systems are able to fight off large amounts of unfriendly bacteria, we may remain symptom-free. But as soon as the balance tips too far, rogue microbes, pathogens, yeast, and bacteria begin to take hold. According to famed French chemist and biologist Antoine Béchamp, viruses can begin to develop from within, infecting the body to the degree that its internal terrain becomes conducive to their growth. If left unchecked, these intestinal imbalances render the body unable to process waste or assimilate what it needs from even the most life-generating foods. A body thus loaded with toxicity ages prematurely and becomes susceptible to disease.

This understanding of human illness may be the single biggest, longest-standing debate separating holistic and allopathic medicine. Holistic practitioners hold fast to Béchamp's position that "the germ is nothing; the terrain is everything." Modern medicine, meanwhile, holds up Louis Pasteur's "germ theory" as the holy grail: that microbes from an external source invade the body and are the first cause of infectious disease. The age-defying detox method draws from a more holistic understanding of the human body.

I don't believe the two perspectives are necessarily mutually exclusive. While I concur with Béchamp that a clean terrain is not hospitable to pathogens, I also believe that Pasteur's germ theory has merit. Modern physical conditions have left us with internal terrains that even significant tissue cleansing cannot fully restore to perfection. The terrain that would theoretically be completely sovereign against germs would have to be akin to the unadulterated terrain of indigenous peoples living a life of impeccable natural purity.

The modern-day scenario leaves us with a double whammy: 1) a deteriorated lineage that has weakened our physical integrity from day one; and 2) a sea of radiation and chemicals that is practically impossible to escape. This combination of conditions makes it much more difficult for even the most die-hard detox enthusiasts to ensure that their internal terrains are immune to all pathogens. I do think that by striving to create the best milieu we can, we can protect ourselves against many pathogens that would otherwise make us sick and weaken our systems. In this way, it is fully worth the effort. I think these two legendary scientists might actually agree on that!

THE KEY TO LONGEVITY

You can take advantage of the latest medications and modalities to suppress your symptoms, but they are not natural and they have their price. Whether you are twenty-nine or ninety-nine, you will get further by focusing less on how *long* you want to live and more on how *well* you want to live. By the same token, you will become more beautiful by focusing less on how young you want to *look* and more on how young you want to *feel*. Everyday regeneration is the key not only to longevity but also to lasting beauty and vitality.

Remember our core natural law: *To experience the grace and vitality of youth, we must flow with nature, not against it.* Think regeneration, not preservation. Quality, not quantity. Because anything else is an attempt to cheat nature—to obstruct its course—and you want nature on your side!

I love the saying "Look where you're going because you'll go where you're looking." When I make choices for myself today, I ask myself if doing this will bring me closer to the person that I want to be—now and for the rest of my life. The woman I envision is quick, beautiful, wise, loving, funny, rambunctious, and oh so alive! Her age does not define her. Rather, there is a timeless radiance about her. She cherishes the gift of each moment. She is neither brittle nor fearful, but carries herself with youthful grace, with her heart open wide to all that life has to offer. What wisdom does she carry? What choices has she made to remain so vital and youthful? I know that if I wish to become her, I must walk the steps that will become her footsteps.

What about you? As you make your everyday choices, whom do you envision becoming?

The Dilemma of the Flower

While probing deeply into the principles of timeless beauty, I frequently stumbled over a seeming conflict in nature. I refer to it as "the dilemma of the flower." How is it, *I asked myself*, that my intuition tells me that a vastly prolonged natural state of youthfulness is our birthright, and yet I behold the flower that lives, blossoms, and dies even as it remains on the vine? *Then, one day, the answer came through in the most wonderful epiphany:* Each human being is not a flower but a whole garden. *While we have cells that, like flowers, naturally bud, blossom, and die, we are also continually generating new cells (or "blossoms") as the old ones die off—and are thus able to enjoy a period of youthful vitality that vastly exceeds our expectations. Aha—mystery solved!*

RUNNING YOUR ENERGY

As human beings, we have evolved to override many of our instincts with learned behaviors. The problem is that many of these socially programmed behaviors expose us to overstimulation and a chronic over-expenditure of energy. I have come to call this phenomenon "running your energy." If you run your energy carelessly—constantly multitasking, burning calories, colluding in the rat race that keeps your adrenals in a hyperactive state of cortisol and adrenaline output, and generally running yourself ragged—you are accelerating the aging process.

Overstimulation, whether chemical or emotional, is often what triggers this behavior. You can run your energy by consuming too many stimulating, acidic substances, since your body must then channel its energies toward regaining balance. At the same time, mainstream news and entertainment have never been more overstimulating. They evoke great emotions in us, of which we, in our passive state, are largely unaware. Gratuitous, excessive violence, crude behavior, vulgar language, and discordant soundtracks are jarring to our senses, causing great inner energy expenditures. We plug in because we assume it is useful, informative, or entertaining, but much of our mainstream media actually offends our nature, running our energy wastefully and throwing us off center.

Overrunning our energy is *youth-degenerating*, and yet this is how we do almost everything in the modern age. Practically speaking, it's culturally mandated. However, it is possible to counteract this phenomenon in our daily lives. As a working parent of three young children in New York City who is constantly juggling the demands of running a household and a business, I would be a ripe mess if I were always running my energy. Now, you may think I'm self-indulgent, but I will tell you that I do not take meetings or see people before noon. Not even my own mother. My husband will corroborate this, as will my kids, who are happily free to raid the kitchen and do whatever they want until I catch up with them after noon.

Why do I insist on keeping my mornings free? Because I value my life force above all. If I don't honor life in myself, how am I to honor life at all? In my busy life, I do not have time or space for energy vampires—those insidious forces of modern living that would run me dry if I let them. Keeping my mornings sacred allows me the time and space to bring myself back to a state of balance and vitality—essential to being the best wife, mother, leader, teacher, colleague, friend, and human being that I can possibly be.

You don't need to make my self-care hours your self-care hours. Find the time that works best for you, but make sure it's a main course in your day, not a mere garnish! I'm always amazed when people say they don't have time to take care of themselves. I know what can get done in a day. There's time. There's just a lack of focused intent. I wouldn't bother with my youth-regenerating regimen if it didn't work. It allows me to approach the rest of my day with greater stores of energy, focus, and productivity. Instead of running my energy in a blind panic to get it all done, I find I have the mental and physical wherewithal to direct my energies far more efficiently.

How do you run your energy throughout your day? Do you clear time and space for regeneration, or do you let this cultural norm dictate how you manage your life? If you want to reap the profound rewards of timeless beauty and youthfulness, you must make it a top priority.

TODAY'S ELECTROMAGNETIC SOUP

I would be utterly remiss if I failed to address the elephant in the room: our ubiquitous use of cell phones and other electronic devices. We are practically swimming in an electromagnetic soup. The hours we spend on our phones and computers, in our cars, in cities, surrounded by buildings and cell-phone towers, and generally exposed to radiation of all kinds is a real threat to our cellular integrity. We are overheating our tissues, threatening our neurological functions, and quite possibly morphing our DNA. Such unnatural dissonance also impacts the endocrine and nervous systems, which are sensitive to external stimuli.

Studies have suggested that radiation poses a threat to human fertility—specifically, to male fertility. In an Argentinean study by Conrado Avendaño, of Nascentis Medicina Reproductiva, sperm from twenty-nine men ages twenty-six to forty-five was placed under a Wi-Fi-connected laptop or away from the computer. As reported in the journal *Fertility and Sterility*, by the end of the experiment, 25 percent of the sperm under the laptop had stopped moving and 9 percent showed DNA damage, whereas 14 percent of samples kept away from the Wi-Fi stopped moving and just 3 percent suffered DNA damage. The researchers determined that the electromagnetic radiation from the wireless connection must have damaged the semen. If the study's findings were correct and wireless radiation damages semen, what further damage might it be doing to the female reproductive system, and to the life force throughout the body? As we await further studies to come in, it would be foolish to ignore the potentially devastating impacts of the wireless lifestyle on our health.

What can you do if your lifestyle requires wireless activity? Aim to neutralize the damage by making sure that everything else you do is highly alkalinizing. Adopt an alkaline diet, get plenty of sleep and exercise, reduce stress, rebalance with meditations and mindfulness, and get out into nature as much as possible. Even daily walks in a city park will help, as will keeping potted plants in your indoor spaces. Use your devices if you must, but don't let them use you! Step away from them at regular intervals to reset and revitalize your energy.

SEXUALITY

Sexuality is fundamental to all life, and a healthy sexuality is a natural benefit of youth regeneration. But in our culture, rather than honoring our sexuality as a healthy and beautiful agent of human connection, we have come to treat it as something demoralizing and warped. So much of our fear of aging is a fear of sexual irrelevance. As long as we are sexually desirable according to the projected cultural standards, we tell ourselves, we will have a valued position in society. We must remain sexy at all costs, otherwise we risk devaluation and isolation. So we do whatever it takes to "look the part," even if it defies nature.

The men I work with are just as concerned about their youth quotient as women. More than ever, men are consciously searching for the lifestyle tools to keep them looking and functioning in their prime. The age of Viagra has revealed that premature diminishing virility is widespread in men and that they are desperate for solutions. You see, men are not so different from women in today's culture. If women measure themselves by their youthfulness and beauty quotient, men measure themselves by their virility quotient. Most of today's women and men were not initiated into the sexual arts in a natural, nurturing, healthy way. We are the products of a culture mired in commercialism, addiction, and pornography. We absorb and carry these imbalanced sexual directives with us throughout our lives. I have found that very few women can say they have a truly healthy body image, and that very few men can say they have a truly healthy attitude toward sex. This is a very sad state of affairs.

Once we become aware of the cultural factors that feed our sexual imbalances, physically and psychologically, we can start to heal them. I recommend that all men and women do a recapitulation exercise focused solely on sexuality. Go through your earliest memories up until the present and identify all the messages you have received consciously, subconsciously, and unconsciously through cultural programming and subliminal media messages. Consider all the sexual experiences you have had throughout your life. Also consider the conclusions you've come to about sexuality, about the opposite sex, and about what it means to be a man or a woman. Determine how those impressions have impacted your relationships, both romantic and platonic. Which ones support your sexual vitality in a healthy way, and which ones counteract or distort it?

If you are concerned about having a weak or even nonexistent libido (sex drive), a common concern in the modern age, it's important to consider all the possible reasons for this. The good news is that it's not merely

Your "Golden Urn"

Internal tonification is a marker of youth, whereas slackness is a marker of degeneration. Taoism, one of the most ancient philosophies we have on record that gives explicit instructions for living in sync with nature, warns of the slackness and prolapse of the internal organs. Among the many sage Taoist traditions is a way of determining internal youthfulness by the tightness of the "golden urn"—or, in Sanskrit, the mula bandha. *We know it in English as the perineum, and for women this includes the perineum and the vaginal opening as a singular composite. It is also well known as the root chakra. A tight but elastic perineum is an indicator of a well-toned set of internal glands and organs. The opposite would indicate prolapsed, slack internal tissues and organs and poorly functioning glands—in short, the kind of system common to modern aging. You can expect the integrity of your "golden urn" to strengthen as you apply the youth-regenerating principles.*

a function of growing older. We should all be able to enjoy a healthy sex life throughout our long lives. But when we consider the way most people typically eat, live, and medicate themselves today, is it any wonder that we're compromising our capacity for sexual joy? How can a body laden with chemical imbalances and obstructions be fully receptive to physical stimulation? If we are getting little sleep, consuming large quantities of acidic foods and substances, calcifying our bodies, accumulating stress, and aging prematurely, is it really so surprising that men and women alike are finding less pleasure in the bedroom?

The good news is that age-defying detox practices help to revive sexual health along with general physical health. A healthy sex life is all about free-flowing conductivity and abundant life force. As you heal your body on the cellular level and remove obstructions to open up your body's pathways, you can expect to experience a wonderful boost in your sexuality!

THE AGING BRAIN

From the allopathic medical perspective, the ravages of brain tissue observed in patients with dementia, Alzheimer's, and other brain diseases are perceived to be the natural wear and tear of an aging brain. However, the holistic health perspective tells quite a different story. If the body, as a whole system, is exposed to substances that undermine any part of it, eventually the rest of the system will be harmed by that initial exposure. To state it another way, the deterioration of the liver, kidneys, blood, lymph, and tissues due to unnatural substances and years of accumulated waste will eventually manifest in the brain. So you can bet the plaque, lesions, and proteins found in the brains of Alzheimer's patients are linked to the plaque, lesions, and proteins found in their hearts, intestines, mouths, and endocrine glands.

What about the genetic connection, you ask? The fact is, we must all pay the price for the missteps of our ancestors. Their mistakes affected the integrity of their DNA coding. We have inherited this degenerated DNA. Parents pass the deteriorated integrity along to their progeny; hence, we see similarly expressing diseases among family members. This is true for every category of acute disease, including dementia. The best way to keep our brains clear and sharp is no different from the best way to stay youthful and beautiful and ward off other forms of degeneration: by syncing up with nature. Break up calcification. Flush out toxins. Maintain freely conducting pathways. Bring abundant oxygen and life force to all of the body's cells.

In addition to this, we know of certain substances that pose a particular threat to the brain: aluminum, mercury, and fluoride. Aluminum and mercury are known neurotoxins, listed as such by the US Environmental Protection Agency (EPA), and yet they are used widely in vaccines and food additives (and, until recently, in dental fillings). Like mercury, aluminum can cross over the blood-brain barrier and build up in the brain over time. Mercury and aluminum have been found in higher quantities in the brains of Alzheimer's patients than in healthy brains—suggesting a clear causal link. While they may help to preserve food and vaccines, they don't do such a good job of preserving brain tissue.

Let this knowledge inspire you to make every effort you can to remove the stores of these poisons from the body through tissue cleansing, and to prevent them from entering your body. If you educate yourself about these lurking offenders, you can make educated choices that resonate with you. Personally, I will never take a flu shot and I don't recommend vaccines—an unpopular choice that can trigger debate, but one that is informed by my research and personal and professional experience.

Fluoride is also used widely in our culture, even though it is also a known poison. Look on any container of rat poison and you'll find the key ingredient listed there is sodium fluoride, which is also in toothpaste and municipal tap water. There is a reason why tubes of toothpaste come with the warning not to ingest it and to keep it out of the reach of children. There may be a higher dosage of fluoride in rat poison, but rats are smaller and we humans use the substance repeatedly throughout the day, every day—especially if we're regularly drinking fluoridated tap water. According to the FluorideAlert.org, "In the past three decades, over 100 studies have found that fluoride exposure can damage the brain." Even low levels of fluoride have been found to harm brain development and been linked to dementia. This is why I avoid tap water and brush with fluoride-free toothpaste.

HORMONE REPLACEMENT THERAPY

Hormone replacement therapy is based on the theory that replacing hormones that are no longer naturally produced in the same quantities after a certain stage of life can prolong the qualities of youth. This is understandably a very attractive prospect; however, it's not as simple as that. HRT is not the youth serum it has been promoted to be. The verdict around the safety and efficacy of HRT is mixed.

When the synthetic version of HRT (typically a blend of estradiol, a version of estrogen, and progesterone), mainly derived from pregnant horse urine, was deemed a precursor of breast and ovarian cancers for women, bioidentical HRT took the spotlight, promising all the benefits of HRT without any of the safety concerns. Bioidentical hormones are considered identical in molecular structure to the hormones women's bodies make. They are synthesized into the identical hormones from plant sources (typically yam and soy). That claim remains dubious—not only because bioidentical hormones have not been proven to be unequivocally safe by longitudinal studies, but moreover because women are entering menopause in chaotic hormonal states from decades of mistreating their bodies. They don't even know how their bodies would have functioned and aged if they had lived with their natural hormonal cycles.

My professional experience and interviews with a vast assortment of women who have unsuccessfully put their hopes in bioidentical HRT supports my general philosophy not to try to trick the body with hormones. Hormones are sacred, as is the endocrine system that secretes them. The body is not easily fooled but is easily aggravated by unnatural treatments. Externally administered hormones do not operate in the same way that naturally secreted hormones do.

Our endocrine glands secrete hormones into our bloodstream, using a complex feedback system that externally administered hormones can disrupt. The pituitary gland and hypothalamus carefully regulate the endocrine hormones' production and secretion. HRT attempts to defy nature by side-stepping this delicate balancing system. While "natural" hormone replacement is very popular today, I disagree with the suggestion that this approach is truly natural or identical. It may be designed in a way that replicates the chemicals in a laboratory, but if I have learned anything over the years, it's that nature cannot be replicated exactly or defied by something manufactured.

Let's peel back another layer and ask why modern women are suffering so much from menopause. The intensity of menopausal symptoms, as with menstrual symptoms, reflects the extent to which the female body must fight to rebalance itself. In the same way that girls in indigenous cultures did not suffer from the modern discomforts of puberty (painful menstruation, acne, moodiness, etc.), historically, indigenous women did not have hot flashes, depression, violent mood swings, and other agonizing symptoms as they experienced menopause. Women were initiated into this stage of life with a new leadership role that afforded them greater admiration and trust. Imagine actually being buoyed by menopause!

Accumulated toxicity is the cause of the discomfort. The more cleanly we live, the more uneventful menopause will be (and, for women of child-bearing years, the more uneventful the menstruation cycle will be). Up until recently, it was only women of the Western world who experienced the discomforts of menopause; there was not even a word for "hot flashes" in Japan! The same is true of osteoporosis (in fact, in cross-cultural research of menopausal women, it has been noted that while estrogen levels dropped in indigenous women, there was not a subsequent rise in bone fractures), not to mention the litany of other terrible female diseases of the reproductive organs, such as endometriosis, polycystic ovary syndrome (PCOS), and fibromyalgia. These are symptoms of imbalanced living, not a factor of living longer. In my practice, I see women experiencing these imbalances as early as in their twenties.

And let's not forget the epic underactive thyroid. Nearly every woman over thirty I have worked with during the past several years has been medicated for a thyroid disorder. Many already had part or all of their thyroid removed by the time they came to see me. The thyroid gland is located in the neck, below the Adam's apple and wrapped around the trachea (windpipe).

This endocrine gland is responsible for secreting many hormones that regulate everything from blood pressure to the rate that food is converted into energy. In my experience, by the time the thyroid registers an imbalanced output of hormones in a blood test, the individual has already spent at least a decade overstimulating the pineal and adrenal glands. This is to say nothing of the pancreas, also a part of the endocrine system, which spends decades overwhelmed with insulin production due to excessive consumption of sugars and starches.

It is the nature of systems that if one or more parts of a system are thrown out of balance, all parts of the system become imbalanced, and nowhere is this better illustrated than in the endocrine system. The endocrine glands are referred to as a system because they are truly part of a whole unit. The seven glands are the pineal, pituitary, thyroid, thymus, pancreas, adrenal, and the testes/ovaries.

Visual stimulation such as from media, computers, video games, flashing neon, and other artificial lights overstimulate the pineal gland (also known as the master gland). Being excessively stressed, which is now a commonly accepted state of being, from grade-school age onward, causes adrenal imbalances. In my practice, I find that everyone with a thyroid imbalance (which expresses as an underactive thyroid or hypothyroid condition) has experienced excessive exposure to these stimuli. However, this is not the only cause; it's also linked with imbalances caused by a low-quality diet and pharmaceutical drugs, and the thyroid can be depleted if a woman has had multiple children.

Many of the women I work with who dedicate themselves to the age-defying detox protocol are eventually taken off the synthetic thyroid replacement drug (usually Synthroid). The few who have had to maintain decreased dosages of Synthroid are the ones who have had their thyroid removed. When this is not enough, a specific form of iodine called nascent iodine can be used. It works wonders to restore the thyroid quickly and effectively! Nascent iodine could be categorized as a precursor to thyroid hormones.

You might be surprised how supportive your doctor will be about decreasing your dose and eventually taking you off the drug completely as your system rebalances and no longer requires the synthetic hormone. When my first group of women reported that their doctors agreed it was time to end the supplementation of Synthroid, we all rejoiced together. I've seen clients work with their doctors to wean off just about every pharmaceutical drug you can imagine as their bodies rebalanced. To the credit of these enlightened, open-minded physicians, they were delighted to help their patients get off their meds, and appreciated the role that cleansing played in their healing. These doctors have often responded by sending me more of their patients!

If you are considering HRT, the question to ask yourself is why? This brings our whole cultural programming around women, beauty, and youth into question. Why are we opposing nature in this way? Beyond the hormonal shifts that come with age are the cultural attitudes toward maturing women. In traditional indigenous cultures, an older woman was highly venerated at this stage of the life cycle, for she was perceived to be taking her place as a wizened mentor to younger generations. She became the story-keeper, the beloved grandmother of the clan. She was not at risk of being abandoned or discarded—not by a long shot! This grandmother represented the clan's most profound ambitions: nobility, wisdom, grace, poise, experience. After a lifetime of being one of the girls, she became a queen.

What would happen if we honored postmenopausal women today as our ancestors did? How would we perceive our womanhood differently if we knew our best years were not behind us? What might we be able to offer younger generations that our image-obsessed culture never could? No amount of HRT will make up for a woman's lack of self-respect. We must earn the venerated perch of feminine nobility, not squander our days worshipping at the altar of youth, chasing commercial notions of beauty, and slaving away to keep up with the Kardashians. If we want to step into a noble role, we must live nobly and pursue noble goals. We must stop fighting nature at every turn and embrace our evolving roles in the life cycle.

By doing this, we can let go of so much fear: the fear of infertility, the fear of diminishment, the fear of irrelevance. Some of us may still choose to color our hair or wear push-up bras—but less out of fear than out of self-love, in the spirit of adornment. Then again, some of us may let nature color our hair and shape our bodies naturally. Either way, when we honor ourselves at every age, fear gives way to self-respect and joyful expression.

In my quest to get to the bottom of the HRT debate, I've spoken with many postmenopausal women in their fifties, sixties, seventies, eighties, and nineties. In addition to interviewing them on the subject of hormone replacement, I analyzed their lives in minute detail to determine the secrets of their success. Many of these women are rare beacons who embody true vitality and joy. What they told me inspired me and supported my theories about the power of syncing up with nature. All of these beautiful, wise, empowered women who have triumphed into their seventies, eighties, and nineties have several key characteristics in common:

- They pivot their lives around a dedicated spiritual framework.

- They live from a place of inspiration, and greet each day with a sense of personal purpose.

- They take excellent care of their bodies, enjoying exceptional nutrition and intestinal health.

- They exercise regularly without "running their energy."

- They prioritize sleep, and are generally early to bed and early to rise.

- They continually give and receive love from friends and family, and do not suffer life-deteriorating relationships.

- They are intellectually curious, eager to read and learn as much as they can about the subjects that captivate them.

- They drink little if any alcohol, and use pharmaceutical drugs sparingly.

- They engage very little in mainstream media.

- They express themselves without hesitation, staying true to themselves and to their visions.

Many women are curious about hormone therapy. In my extensive interviews with women who have opted for HRT, there is not one of them who is better off for it over the long term. The ones that took bioidenticals were either unimpressed with them or disappointed, and soon went off them. Each concluded that HRT was not the answer, though several felt there was some benefit to natural progesterone cream periodically. Their logic was to try it and see if it helped. As we know, different things work for different people. If it is clearly not working for you in a tangible, visible, meaningful way, don't let the theoretical information sway you. (If you want to read further on this subject, I recommend *What Your Doctor May Not Tell You about Menopause* by Dr. John R. Lee. It's most illuminating!)

When it comes to HRT, bioidentical or otherwise, I believe that women should be properly educated first and then given the freedom to weigh the risks and choose what resonates with them. However, any path that opposes nature or tries to outsmart it will lead to many obstructions along the way before the final stop. My advice? Chase the illusion of youth at your own peril, or else start cultivating the real thing! Beauty flows from inner health. If we cleanse our systems, increase conductivity, deepen our flexibility, and strengthen our connections with the greater community of life, our internal rhythms will naturally self-correct. But we have to appreciate the depth of the cleansing required and be patient, trusting that this is how true beauty and youthfulness can manifest at any age.

The Natural Progesterone Cream Caveat
Although I am not a fan of bioidentical hormone replacement in general, sometimes a woman experiences a bit of estrogen dominance caused by prolonged nursing, overexposure to environmental estrogens, too much adipose tissue (fat and estrogen feed one another), and various other reasons. In such cases, and provided she has stopped breastfeeding, a woman may opt to purchase a tube of natural progesterone cream at the health-food store and apply it sparingly to the soft tissue (inner thighs, inner arms, neck) twice daily for the second fourteen days of her cycle each month for one to three months, or as otherwise instructed by a trusted health-care professional. The cream can be used as a bridge when combined with deep-tissue cleansing to help rebalance the hormones and prevent the condition from snowballing. But it should not be used for a prolonged period, as it may trigger further hormone imbalances.

You know that there's a serious endocrine imbalance when you see someone "of a certain age" whose gender is no longer clearly discernible. Have you ever noticed an older man start to develop breasts and hips, or a woman become shapeless with facial hair? What is this all about? A life lived insulting the endocrine glands can result in this midlife gender-hormone fallout.

Estrogen dominance is the most common hormone imbalance, affecting both men and women of every age. This is because our environment has become overly estrogenic. Environmental estrogens are in everything from carpets to detergents, from pesticides to plastics and nonstick cookware. These hormone disrupters are responsible for cancer, reproductive problems, and mood disorders—to name just a few. It is virtually impossible to avoid all of these things in the modern world, but we can reduce our exposure to them as much as possible by eating foods grown without pesticides, avoiding plastics, using natural cookware and cleaning products, and outfitting our homes and bodies with organic fabrics.

There are many symptoms of estrogen dominance. According to one of the most renowned hormone doctors, the late Dr. John R. Lee (www.john leemd.com), estrogen dominance accelerates aging and causes breast cancer, allergies, fat gain, depression, decreased libido, insomnia, memory loss, infertility, and much more.

Over age fifty, men should still look like men and women should still look distinctly like women. If your appearance makes you suspect an endocrine imbalance in yourself, or if you want to prevent it from happening, there is only one safe and natural solution: Get serious about cellular cleansing in order to give your endocrine system a chance to rebalance itself.

BONES BUILT TO LAST

Our bones are built to last. Deterioration of the bones—such as in the case of osteoporosis, where bones become porous, brittle, and subject to fracture—is simply an effect of demineralization. This demineralization is due to over-consumption of acidifying foods, drinks, medications, and other substances, and the accumulation of their waste residues. The bones are the most alkaline part of the body, so the worst thing we can do for them is consume large amounts of acidic substances. When we do this, our blood becomes acidic and leaches alkalinity, in the form of calcium, from the bones to prevent organ damage throughout the system. The good news is that we can take the following steps to re-mineralize our bones and our teeth:

- Alkalinize the diet.

- Remove internal obstructions to support the flow of alkaline blood in the body's pathways.

- Get plenty of sunlight for vitamin D, the unparalleled nutrient for healthy bones and teeth!

We begin by removing the acidifying substances from our diet/lifestyle. In addition to obvious offenders (cigarettes; alcohol; caffeine; chemicals; sugary, starchy, oily, processed foods, etc.), we must steer clear of carbonated beverages—and not just sodas. Carbonated mineral water has come to be widely accepted as a healthy choice, but this could not be further from the truth. Any carbonated drink introduces carbonic acid to the body (which already has too much of it from shallow breathing and poor digestion) and contributes to the excessive gas pressure in the body. Where does this gas pressure go as it accumulates? It gets pushed deeper in the bones and tissues, further weakening the bones. The bones do not want to share space with gas, but because they are porous, the gas finds space to land in them.

We must also consume the best-quality alkalinizing foods we can find. Begin with organic, dark leafy green vegetables, particularly via juicing. If there is one thing you can do immediately to regenerate your bones, it is juicing organic leafy greens. Then, we remove the accumulation of acidic waste matter and its acidic by-products from the intestine. And we mustn't forget to seek out plenty of vitamin D through daily exposure to sunlight.

When we eat and cleanse for bone health, we feel it in our bones. We feel stronger and better supported. Every part of the body has a corresponding emotional connection. Bone trouble is linked to a lack of support. If you suffer from weak bones, consider whether you lack support in one or several areas of your life, and make the necessary adjustments.

> ### Tune In to Your Bones
> *Think of your skeletal system as a crystalline transistor. Your bones are made of minerals that conduct information in the same way rock transmits the currents of the Earth's pulsations throughout the planet. Like crystals, your bones hold information and memory. Take a moment to think about all that implies and then give praise to your skeletal system for its remarkable design. Take another balanced breath when you are ready, and imagine your entire bone network filled with light: a powerful golden-white glow—clear and strong. Feel the current of this blissful vibration moving through your bones and radiating throughout your entire body. Notice your feet and the hundreds of tiny bones that support you. Now picture the earth beneath your feet. As you set your feet upon the lovely texture of rich dirt, imagine roots reaching from the bones in your feet like vines pouring into the soft earth, making you feel supported and connected. Meld your energy with the fertile terrain. Honor the conductive power of your skeletal system!*

HEALTHY TEETH

Like bones, teeth are made up of calcium, phosphorous, and other minerals, and are vulnerable to acidity. We think of bacteria as the primary cause of tooth decay, but the precursor to bacteria is acidity. Acidic foods stick in the cells and tissues, blocking the flow of life force in the body and thus signaling bacteria to break down the nonviable matter. Bacteria are just doing their job by appearing in the mouth and proceeding to eat away the tooth and gums. The mouth is the first line of defense against acidic substances, so if you have lots of cavities, consider that as a heads-up that your bones are next in line. Cavity-free teeth are the result of a healthy whole-body system.

All of the fat-soluble vitamins—but particularly vitamins K2, A, and D—are essential for preventing and reversing tooth decay. However, supplementation is not as effective as receiving these vitamins in their whole-food form (or from pure sunshine, as in the case of vitamin D). The best sources of vitamins K2 and A are animal organs, which, understandably, you may find unappetizing. Although I encourage you to explore whether this approach may be helpful for you (particularly if you don't intend to undertake significant, long-term cellular cleansing), I generally don't recommend consuming animal organs for these vitamin needs. It requires killing more animals and ingesting their toxicity.

I'm not a fan of fish liver oil, even though decades ago such a protocol may have been safer when our oceans were less toxic. Remember, the liver is the organ that processes heavy toxicity. Do you really want the oil from modern fish liver? But don't despair. If you balance and detoxify your body through deep cellular cleansing, it will regenerate what it needs. If you are concerned that the cleansing process will take too long and you have dire teeth issues that cannot wait, here are the foods that are high in fat-soluble vitamins and less toxic to our bodies:

- Pure organic ghee and butter

- Raw egg yolks

- Cold-pressed olive oil

If I were working to reverse tooth decay or bone loss, I would drink two ounces of fresh wheatgrass juice four to six days a week. In the meantime, I would pepper my diet with ghee, raw butter, and hard raw goat cheeses—all of which have a place in the detox method. Wheatgrass, fresh sprouts, and dark leafy greens provide the highly alkaline, mineral-rich substances the teeth and bones require for repair and maintenance in the modern world that supplements in pill form cannot.

As for vitamin D, it's all in the sun's rays. Do not underestimate the healing power of the sun! The cleaner we become, and the more aligned with nature's electromagnetic currents, the more we can conduct the sun's healing rays without toxic sunscreens. This is assuming, of course, that we exercise common sense and sun ourselves only in the safe morning and late-afternoon hours.

However, here's another caveat: There is nothing more acidic than computer and cell-phone radiation, so if your body is busy trying to keep its bloodstream alkaline while you're on your computer and smartphone all day and living in a city (hello, that's me!), you will still be vulnerable to the modern triggers of demineralization throughout your body. These methods will just help you to neutralize some of that acidity and thereby reduce the damage. The only way to ensure perfect bone and tooth health is to choose another way to live.

For the record, I haven't had a single cavity since I adopted the cleansing lifestyle fifteen years ago; before that, I would get the occasional cavity even though I brushed several times a day with fluoridated toothpaste. Cavities are a crisis of the civilized world.

SLEEP REGENERATION

In our culture, we think of sleep much as we think of water. We are told that we need eight hours of sleep and eight glasses of water each day, but we rarely give our daily requirements of rest and hydration much more thought than that. We keep the number eight in mind as a benchmark, but we don't take it seriously until we get serious about improving our health or losing weight. Nor do we think much about the quality of our sleep, which is just as critical as the quality of our waking lives. Just as eight glasses of water a day is not going to help you much if you are subsisting on a diet of soda, burgers, and fries, eight hours of sleep is not going to help much if your days are overly stressful and you must rely on sleeping aids to power down.

So let's get past this superficial recommendation of eight hours of sleep and understand what sleep is really about. Getting quality sleep is mandatory for youth regeneration. It is also one of the most powerful ways to sync up with nature. Nature runs on cycles and rhythms. The sleep cycle is a multifaceted clockwork interlinked with critical hormone secretion and organ renewal. (Just consider the madness of anti-aging hormone therapy in the context of running our energy and getting too little sleep!) The circadian rhythm is the master clock of the body. It works with and governs all of the rhythms in the body, including the digestive and reproductive cycles. If you oppose your body's natural rhythms with too much artificial stimulation (e.g., from acidic foods, drugs, entertainment, computer screens, stress, etc.), you rob yourself of your innate powers of self-renewal.

Thanks to ancient Chinese and Ayurvedic texts, we know a great deal about what goes on during the night to recharge us. According to these sources, the body functions like clockwork; when you are deep in sleep, your liver can detoxify and repair between eleven p.m. and midnight; your small intestine can process waste between two and six a.m.; and the large intestine can remove waste between six a.m. and noon. These same sources concur that all the while, the endocrine system is balancing and secreting its powerful hormones into the blood, regulating all the systems of the body. If you are suffering from any imbalance, I suggest reflecting on your sleep patterns and finding ways to prioritize proper sleep in your life. I'll tell you what I tell my clients: Sleep as if your life (not only youthfulness) depends on it—because it does!

La cure de sommeil is French for the sleep cure, which can be done at home, on vacation, or at a clinic. The idea is that by sleeping for many hours longer than usual (in sleep clinics, this can be up to twenty hours a day for ten to twelve days), the body can do its best healing. How many of us (parents of multiple young children, especially) would love to check ourselves into a clinic to sleep for ten days? There are times when I can't think of a better way to spend a vacation! When we're sleeping we're not consuming, we're not being stimulated, and we are not expending. We are simply at rest on nature's operating table, being renewed.

For many people, finding the time to sleep is not the problem; it's being able to fall asleep at an appropriate hour. Insomnia and restlessness are co-factors of a life of overstimulation and overexpending one's energy. If you harmonize your waking hours with your natural circadian rhythms, sleep will come naturally. Taking the following steps can help tremendously:

- Remove all sources of artificial light in your sleeping space (e.g., cover or turn off the radio alarm clock, draw curtains against neon lights from outside, remove or turn off your smartphone).

- Take a bath before bed (or a shower if that's all you have access to) with the conscious directive to remove negative energy accumulated from the day.

- Make a list of all the things on your mind to do the following day and then set it aside for the morning, so that stressful thought patterns do not interfere with your path to restful sleep.

- Remind yourself that in sleep you will gain the energy you need to undertake tomorrow's demands skillfully and elegantly.

- If there is a problem troubling you, remind yourself that when you wake from a restful sleep, you will have the clarity of mind to solve it.

- Identify where you may be holding negative energy in your body. Take a deep breath, and on the exhale, release the energy; then fill the space with peace. Do this as many times and in as many parts of your body as necessary to calm your whole body and invite sleep.

As with fasting, when you regenerate your system with sleep, you will notice that you are not gaining more energy and improving organ function by taking in superfoods or miracle powders. The revitalization comes from less stimulation and less expenditure of energy. You are allowing your body to reactivate its brilliant self-healing design and, ultimately, to reconnect with the grid of living energy continually flowing all around it. Sleep because your life depends on it, and also because it's essential for lasting beauty.

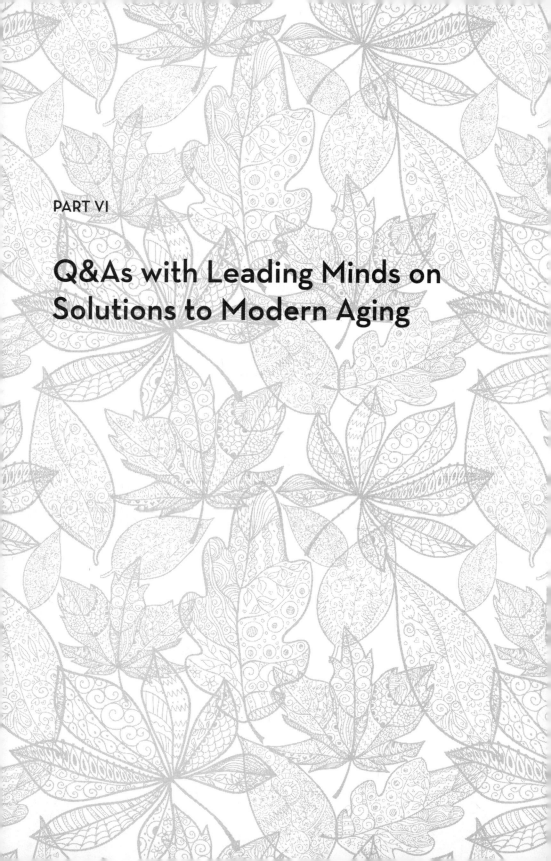

PART VI

Q&As with Leading Minds on Solutions to Modern Aging

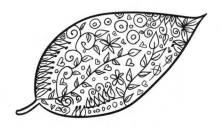

I n a world buzzing with a great deal of chatter about health and rejuvenation, there are a few notable experts who meld their unstoppable passion and enthusiasm for the topic with deep clinical and medical knowledge. From these individuals we can glean the most advanced information on modern aging solutions available today. I have had the distinct pleasure and honor of interviewing seven of these leading health practitioners—two MDs, two PhDs, an ND, a certified researcher of biological medicine, and a raw-food chef. I hope you find these interviews to be as immensely enjoyable and enlightening as I have.

You will see that their messages share much in common, such as the promise of vigorous longevity when the body is allowed to rebalance and regenerate in a healthy environment. But there are also conflicting opinions among these experts, particularly around the integration of bioidentical hormones. I recommend using these interviews as a launching pad for your own self-education. Let the various perspectives inspire you to learn more and discover what resonates most strongly for you.

While the opinions and protocols offered in the following interviews do not always align perfectly with mine, they do all inform and broaden our understanding of youth regeneration, which is why I feel it is important to share them all—no holds barred. So herewith, I present seven of the finest minds on the topic of solutions to modern aging: Dr. Eric Braverman, Dr. Jon Turk, Dr. Sherrill Sellman, Dr. Fred Bisci, Richard Harvey, Mimi Kirk, and Tonya Zavasta.

Q&A WITH DR. ERIC BRAVERMAN

Dr. Eric Braverman, an MD in integrative and internal medicine, is the director of the Place for Achieving Total Health (PATH) in New York City and the former chief clinical researcher at the Princeton Brain Bio Center. Dr. Braverman is the best-selling author of several books on anti-aging, diet, and brain health, including *Younger You, The Younger (Thinner) You Diet, Younger (Sexier) You,* and *Younger Brain, Sharper Mind.*

You're only as young as your oldest part.

—Dr. Eric Braverman

NR: Tell me about the philosophy of your practice.
EB: People are aging very fast. Thirty- to forty-year-olds are waiting for sections of their body to break down; then the medical companies can make money on it. Generally, for women, the first part to break down are the ovaries and the bones and muscles. An inadequate frame leads to brain instability, which leads to a host of neuropsychological problems: anxiety, depression, memory problems, etc. People have an overly emotional view of aging. Women take all of this into their relationships, to their spouses and boyfriends or other relationships. Men have their own imbalances, but this is what happens with women. The reason men are attracted to women in their twenties is because of their physical and emotional optimism. They can't have real intimacy with these twenty-somethings, but this is what drives older men to younger women. It's not because the younger women are more attractive. By repairing a woman's system so she can have all the value of her maturity and also radiate that physical and emotional optimism, she can have it all.

NR: Do you recommend HRT/bioidentical hormones?
EB: Around thirty years of age a woman's estrogen production begins to decline, and by forty most women need mild hormonal repair. I only use bioidentical hormone replacement therapy. By forty we will already see

changes in a woman's memory, sleep, ability to process mentally; we see a dramatic decline in her muscle tone (the average body fat among my patients is 32 percent; ideal body fat for women is about 22 percent) and skeletal frame. Of course we also see a big change in sexuality and addictions. In my practice, a patient begins with a full medical checkup: physical and cognitive. Based on this, I will give her an ideal protocol of growth hormone DHEA, testosterone, estrogen, thyroid, sleep, and blood sugar support, and memory enhancement aids.

NR: Do you find that all women need all of this?
EB: Need is an interesting word. It all depends on their goals. If someone wants to live to one hundred and look and feel fifty (if we can pretend there's a net-zero aging), that person will need to undertake the full protocol. A woman at thirty or forty who repairs herself will get another ten to fifteen years of vigor. By age fifty-five, a huge number of people have already lost a significant amount of muscle and bone, are sleeping poorly, have some degree of depression or moodiness, and are precancerous. I can give them twenty-five things for their internal repair. They will do twenty-five things in an evening to get ready to go out (get dressed, put on makeup, adorn themselves with jewelry, dress their partner to match, etc.). They will just as easily do these things I give them to do for their internal repair.

NR: Do you find that someone who has taken care to eat a healthy diet, sleep, exercise, and lead a low-stress natural life ages differently than your average patient?
EB: A good diet can add seven more years to your life. Taking care of your mind, your cognitive well-being, can add another seven years. Sleeping well can add another seven to ten years. And keeping thin and fit can add another ten to fifteen years. You can add forty years to your life in terms of your medical capacity by prioritizing these things.

To learn more about Dr. Braverman's practice, visit http://pathmed.com.

Q&A WITH DR. JON TURK

Dr. Jon Turk is a respected facial plastic surgeon with practices in Manhattan and Long Island. He was voted one of the top surgeons of New York by his peers and recognized as one of America's Best Doctors by *New York* magazine. For individuals seeking facial rejuvenation without surgery, he provides a wealth of nonsurgical skin-care options.

The minute you do something that looks "done" is the minute you've defeated the purpose of having something done.

—Dr. Jon Turk

NR: What is the average age that men and women respectively decide to have work done to make them look younger?
JT: It used to be that the average patient was in the sixty to sixty-five range; fifties for an eye lift; sixty to seventy for a face-lift. But with the advent of injectables and fillers, we started to see both men and women coming in much earlier because these methods were much less invasive. The trend shifted down toward fifty. Now with our new prevention tools, the trend is shifting even younger—to forty. There are even a number of thirty-somethings who come in to formulate a beauty strategy that begins with collagen stimulation.

NR: What are these new prevention tools, and how do they work?
JT: The new prevention methods are really part of a paradigm shift in how plastic surgeons view their patients. For a long time we did things reactively. We would undertake to fix things once they happened; now we can prevent loss of elasticity and collagen and influence regeneration. This creates a whole different field, putting aside cutting, pulling, and injecting by manipulating the body's own remarkable ability to heal itself. The old era was the era of injectables from animals and synthetics. The new era is about enabling collagen to be reconfigured from within.

NR: What are these minimally invasive procedures?
JT: There are several procedures that safely and predictably regenerate collagen and stimulate elasticity and circulation, resulting in younger-looking
skin. Dermapen is a minimally invasive procedure that uses a completely
natural plant-based lubricant with a mechanical device to micro-needle
the skin. This has no adverse effect; it simply creates controlled surface and
subsurface wounds that trick the body into stimulating collagen naturally,
strengthening and thickening the stratum corneum (the outermost layer
of the epidermis) and improving microcirculation. Next there is Exilis,
which uses radio frequency energy to tighten and remodel the dermis and
increases the turnover of collagen. This is something that works great for
anyone aged thirty-five to sixty-five. Finally, we have Selphyl platelet injections, or PRP, which stands for platelet-rich plasma. The patient's platelets
are extracted from a small tube of their own blood and reinjected into the
face, stimulating collagen, elastin, and improved circulation to the skin.

*NR: How long do the effects of these procedures last, and how much do
they cost?*
JT: The effects of a series of sessions (usually three to four sessions) will
last about one to two years. Maintenance is recommended on a monthly to
yearly basis, depending on the procedure. Fees range from $500 to $1,500
per session, again depending on the procedure, with the full cost of an
initial treatment program ranging between $1,500 and $2,500.

NR: What is your stance on hormone replacement therapy?
JT: The main issue with estrogen loss is diminished collagen production.
Diminished collagen results in dryness, lack of elasticity, and a general
lack of the luster that makes skin look youthful. However, estrogen is only
one part of the equation. Just because a postmenopausal woman is taking
a form of estrogen doesn't mean her skin is going to look youthful. There
are many other factors involved, and in my experience, the biggest things
that impact the appearance of the skin and the skin's ability to respond to

any procedures are alcohol, sun exposure, and tobacco. You can feel the difference in elasticity in a woman's skin if she drinks (even socially, but without proper balance), smokes, and has overexposed herself to the sun. The results of the same operation or procedure can be vastly different based on these factors. That said, if there were a safe way to replace estrogen, it would have a very beneficial effect on the skin.

To learn more about Dr. Jon Turk, visit www.jonturkmd.com.

Q&A WITH DR. SHERRILL SELLMAN

Dr. Sherrill Sellman is a naturopathic doctor, author, radio host, and international lecturer. She is the author of *Hormone Heresy* and *What Women Must Know to Protect Their Daughters from Breast Cancer*. I was fortunate to be able to interview her at length about hormonal balance in women as it pertains to regenerating beauty and youthfulness.

Menopause is kind of a magnified experience of how well the body is functioning in general, so we blame a lot of things on menopause, but it really is just the red light on the dashboard, giving us information.
—Dr. Sherrill Sellman

NR: Tell us a little bit about your philosophy pertaining to youth regeneration and hormones.
SS: I'm a naturopathic doctor. I got into this world because of my own hormonal havoc when I was in my forties. It forced me to really learn about my body, learn about hormones, address underlying issues that were causing my hormones to be out of balance—and also to uncover many myths and misinformation, which really fuels my passion. As a result of what I was learning, and healing in my own body, I began to write about it, and it led to the creation of my first book, *Hormone Heresy*. I continued to write and research as my journey continued, revealing what it really takes to rejuvenate our hormones as we age in life.

NR: Comparing women who truly care for themselves with greater awareness and those who don't, do you see a difference in how they experience menopause and what happens with their hormones and their endocrine systems?

SS: Oh, absolutely, because hormone imbalance really is a symptom of underlying compromised functioning. Hormones don't just exist out there in space, disconnected from everything else going on in your life, including your thoughts, emotions, spiritual orientation, and perception of reality. Everything is impacting how your body is working. And to the degree you are committing yourself to a healthy, integrated lifestyle, you are going to be supporting your body and its ability to maintain health and balance—especially during major times of transition when the body really requires everything to be firing on all cylinders, so to speak.

So to the degree women are caught up in stress, or in a toxic environment, or eating sugar and carbs and not sleeping properly, or on various medications, and affecting their adrenals in many ways, they are going to have a rougher journey. And not just a rougher journey through menopause. Menopause is kind of a magnified experience of how well the body is functioning in general, so we blame a lot of things on menopause, but it really is just the red light on the dashboard, giving us information. Times of transition just add more stress to the system.

NR: So for women who are taking care of their bodies, is there still some support you can offer?

SS: When we say "taking care of our bodies," it's kind of a generalization, isn't it? When people tell me in my practice that they're eating a good diet, that to me is a meaningless statement unless I have more information about what's going on in their bodies, what their diet really is, what nutrition they're taking in other forms. And also, I do a lot of testing based on their genetic expression, which is called *nutrigenomic testing*.

I can tell you a few things I've learned that have made a huge impact in my practice and benefited my patients. The vast majority of people—I could probably say this of just about every person I've tested—have challenges in dealing with a toxic world. The liver's ability to detox hormones, which is called Phase 1, is severely compromised for just about everybody. So even if we are eating appropriately—cutting down on carbs, and getting lots of good veggies, complex carbs found in veggies and fruits, good sources of protein, and your healthy fats—we are challenged. We haven't evolved genetically to deal with a toxic world without support, and I see this all the time.

This particularly affects how efficient people are at breaking down and eliminating the estrogens—and I'm talking about endocrine-disrupting chemicals, like Bisphenol A (BPA), which everybody has in their bodies (children are born with Bisphenol A), the hormones that we are making each month, and the hormones that we may be taking from the Pill, or from some form of hormone replacement therapy. When we don't have the capacity to properly metabolize and break down these estrogen molecules, they may turn into a more-potent form of a metabolite that the body reabsorbs, stimulating more estrogen levels. The hot flashes, night sweats, PMS, the fibroids, the endometriosis, the weight gain, the risk of cancers—they are all related to high estrogen levels.

Even during our menopausal years, we very rarely find a woman who's truly deficient in estrogen, especially remembering that our fat cells make estrogen, and if women are overweight to any degree, they are generating lots of estrogen. And then if our liver isn't working efficiently, we are increasing exposure to very potent and proliferative estrogen. (Estrogen proliferates cell growth; that's why it's a risk factor for cancer.) This can be a serious problem, including all the symptoms that I just mentioned.

NR: What are your solutions for this?
SS: Well, first of all, you need to eat a diet that is very rich in cruciferous vegetables—broccoli, kale, cauliflower, radishes, arugula, watercress, rutabaga—because this family actually has phytochemicals that support the enzymes that do the job in Phase 1. Everyone should be eating them. However, my caveat about this is, I don't believe you should be eating most of the family (other than maybe arugula, watercress, and radishes) in the

raw form, because they are really hard to break down and digest. I prefer them to be slightly steamed or fermented. That's the best way to ensure you're absorbing and assimilating the active ingredients, because they're very protective in this Phase 1 part of the liver.

The other thing is, I believe most people should be taking a support nutrient supplement that is particularly targeting their ability to detox, and it should include the active ingredients of cruciferous vegetables known as I3C, indole-3-carbinol. Another form of it is called Di-indole Methane, DIM. So if you see a support product that has DIM or I3C, that's really important. You can get other components to a good supplement, but I think that should be a standard part of every woman's health plan, and every man's. (In men there's an increased risk of prostate cancer, which is an estrogen-driven cancer.)

NR: What about using progesterone? How would you integrate progesterone therapy?
SS: When I was in my early forties, my lifestyle, stress, diet—everything took a toll on me. And it was showing up as anxiety attacks at about three or four in the morning. I had this insomnia, then I was getting night sweats, and occasionally hot flashes. I had severe arthritis and severe hay fever. I could go on and on with the litany of symptoms! So when I was looking for help and realized I was dealing with a hormonal thing, I started investigating natural progesterone, and I started using it. That was quite profound because the symptoms—the night sweats, anxiety attacks, most of what we call menopausal symptoms—are actually symptoms that occur in the perimenopausal years. Menopause is twelve complete months without a menstrual cycle.

Generally by the time we have completed twelve months, we're out of the fluctuation and reduction of hormones. Our ovaries reduce estrogen production by 40 to 60 percent, but never totally cease to function, and we have backup systems like our adrenal glands—and also, remember, our fat cells make estrogen. So generally we have this condition called *estrogen dominance*. (We've found this through the most accurate way to assess hormones, saliva testing, not the blood test, which is a flawed test that gives flawed readings. Women need to be aware of this, which is why I've written about this topic extensively in *Hormone Heresy*.) We are showing up with high insulin levels, which generate high estrogen levels, and stress, which creates cortisol.

So what's really happening is that we have an excess and an imbalance—too much estrogen without enough of its balancing hormone, called progesterone. When I learned about this, I tried using progesterone and, literally, within a month, the night sweats and the hot flashes disappeared, my sleep improved—it was phenomenal. And it was really helping to balance the excess of estrogen.

However, I will tell you what I have learned since then. Progesterone is not the be-all and end-all; it is not the magic bullet. It will help support a system that is greatly out of balance, but it will not correct the condition long-term. In order to correct the underlying reasons, we have to address our adrenal glands, which create and support and maintain our hormones, and our hormone balance—especially in our menopausal years. And this is where the big problem lies for all women. We have adrenal exhaustion, and it upsets many systems and functions in the body. Without supporting the adrenals, progesterone taken long-term will not be effective; it will only be effective in the short term, while we're addressing underlying issues.

NR: I'd like to hear more about the adrenals, but first, is there a particular protocol you use for the progesterone? If you use a cream, where do you apply it, and how much?
SS: You apply it topically, in the areas that are well absorbed, which is the soft tissue, like the inner arms, the chest, inner thighs, back of the knees—where your body can absorb it readily. You would apply it in the morning and in the evening. As far as the frequency, it just depends on what's going on with you. Women have used it to help with PMS, with fertility, with hot flashes. It depends on where you are in your life cycle, and what your symptoms are.

But hormones are very powerful substances; you don't just play around with them. The reason why I believe progesterone should be used as part of a protocol and not be relied on long-term is because I have looked at saliva tests of women who have used it long-term, and their levels are excessively high. And if your levels are excessively high, you're going to upset this very delicate hormonal balance, which makes your estrogen levels very low, so it shows up as another range of symptoms, which mimic estrogen deficiency. Hormonal balance is a very delicate thing.

I recommend that if women need some support with progesterone, to do it for three months while addressing and getting other systems back in balance again. It's a temporary support, not a cure-all. I've been doing thousands of saliva tests, and I just see a lot of overdosing of progesterone, and the lab that I work with sees a tremendous amount of tests coming in with women who've been on progesterone for years and are so out of balance that it leads to another range of issues. So use it judiciously. I see it as a way to support yourself *while* you are addressing the deeper issues that drive all these imbalances.

NR: Let's go back to the adrenals. Adrenal fatigue is the root cause, then, of hormonal imbalance?
SS: Yes, adrenal fatigue. I consider it the root cause because the adrenals actually impact how hormones are expressed in the body. What I mean by that is, when you're stressed, making too much cortisol, it can block progesterone receptors; it can impair thyroid receptors; it creates what we call Reverse T3, which blocks the absorption of active thyroid hormones, so you can have a hypothyroid kind of condition. It can increase estrogen production in the body. It raises insulin, which is a fat-storage hormone, and then the more fat we're storing, the more we're making estrogen— so it's a very critical component of hormonal balance. We really need to understand the major role. If you want to rejuvenate your body for the long term, you must support your adrenal glands, nourish and strengthen and, as Chinese medicine would say, "tonify" them, which is a key focus of my own personal protocol, and the protocol I work with in my practice.

NR: What are the top ways to get the adrenals back in balance? I imagine putting the smartphone down before bed would be helpful.

SS: Never have your phone anywhere near your bed—that literally stresses the adrenals. A high-carbohydrate diet is one of the most aging things. We need to use vitamin C, because the adrenals use more vitamin C than any other organ in the body. We need to give our adrenals forms of adaptogen—plants that practitioners of herbal medicine claim decrease cellular sensitivity to stress—such as maka, Siberian ginseng, ashwagandha, or American ginseng—there are numerous adaptogen formulations. B vitamins are really important. Minerals are really important. Most of all, it's important to reduce stress. I can give women all the stuff they want, but if they don't rest and allow themselves to have some downtime, nothing is going to restore those adrenals. That's one of our big challenges.

NR: So it's really about creating a new paradigm.

SS: I talk about this a lot in my book. It's about honoring and healing the feminine, because our patriarchal culture pushes us, and we don't honor the cycles or the needs of our bodies; and we don't appreciate rest and being receptive as much as we value being externalized and active and masculine. That's part of our wound that keeps us in this stressed-out, harmonically imbalanced place.

NR: What is your ideal vision of a woman who's moving into another phase of life? What would that look like?

SS: I want to say something about women who have given birth. I have a lot of faith in the wisdom of traditional Chinese medicine. We have this amazing life force we come in with, but how we live our life determines whether it is saved like a trust fund or squandered. Certainly, after giving birth—because birth is a huge demand on our energies—women need to recuperate and regenerate.

In the traditional Chinese culture, after a woman gave birth, she would have months in confinement. People would come and give her special soups, help with the baby, and let her rest and rejuvenate, because to the degree that she didn't do that she would lose her essences and be more prone to hormonal imbalances, depression, and other issues down the track.

But today we rush back and go shopping with our three-week-old baby! I think, culturally, we really need to understand the role and power of having rest and learning how to say no. We need to make sure we meditate on a daily basis, be in nature on a daily basis, and of course, to get some exercise in. We learn to live in balance by listening to our inner self when it's appropriate to give our energy out and when to hold our energy in and rejuvenate it. And how to move in life with the seasons. Summer is externalized, a high-energy time; winter is a low-energy time, when we're hibernating, rejuvenating, regenerating. So we're learning how to move in balance with all the stages and seasons of our life, to really honor the wisdom of our feminine self—and our intuition, which is our greatest strength. But we need to be quiet and listen in order to have the gift of that intuition readily available to us.

NR: What can a woman who has had children expect to have happen to her body and her endocrine system in her later years?
SS: When you are pregnant, it's a huge, huge energy demand on your body because you're creating another life. It's pulling on your energies, your essences, your nutrition, so you must recover properly from a birth. If you're nursing, again, it's demanding a lot from the body, because you're making all this milk, which requires energy and nutrition.

In Chinese medicine, they don't so much talk about adrenals; what they talk about is kidney energies. This is an energetic system of the body that affects two aspects of ourselves. It affects our energy output, our stamina—not just the energy we use to get through our day, but also the energy to make sure all the systems and functions are able to work optimally. We need energy on a cellular level to make sure we're detoxifying and managing blood sugar and rebuilding. So that's called the *yong*, which is more associated with what we know as adrenals—the dynamic energy that gets us up and going.

Then the other facet is called the *yin*. The *yin* is a more nourishing, lubricating, quieter, calmer, more peaceful energy. If you're deficient in yin, you start experiencing creaky joints, more agitation, impaired sleep, and everything will start drying out—your mucus membranes, your skin, your eyes, your vaginal tissue—which is a big problem I see for women under stress. They are getting very deficient in their *yin*, and also in their *yong*, which means they don't have libido. They're frazzled, they're exhausted. They just take their cups of coffee to keep going because their natural ability to generate energy is really being depleted.

So the key to rejuvenation in the Chinese model is rejuvenating these kidney essences. You do that through diet, lifestyle, meditation, and through specific tonics. The art of Chinese medicine is to use herbs that actually have similar hormonal essences. The Chinese rejuvenate hormones through herbal formulations that have the ability to nourish these glands and systems. That's what I have been using for years. I don't use bioidentical hormones; I'm not particularly a fan of them, because they are only supplementing, not rejuvenating and regenerating our own essences.

You need to regenerate and rejuvenate your essences, starting from the time you're a young woman all the way through life—because the demands only increase as you get pregnant, have children, a job, and a life. This is depleting our essences, and I just see this day in and day out with all the women I work with. They're exhausted, they can't think, their memory is gone, their libido is gone, they have vaginal dryness, they are putting on weight; there are just all these issues that start showing up as symptoms of deficiency. I personally address these issues by working with a Chinese herbalist to personalize natural formulas to rejuvenate these essences. I've seen amazing results. If you can really nourish this part of you, you can stay healthy, balanced, energetic, have good libido, have good, youthful skin, and you can stay that way as you move through those stages of life.

It's a critical component not understood in Western medicine. In Western medicine, if you show up with vaginal dryness (and this is happening to women in their forties because they are so exhausted and depleted), you will be put on estrogen. Well, it will help to restore vaginal tissue, but you are now absorbing estrogen in your body, and not getting to the root cause of why that's happening. You're going to have to use it for the rest of your life—not a good idea.

NR: Would you call these Chinese herbs precursors to the hormones? And are there certain ones that you use most often?
SS: I wouldn't call them precursors; I'd call them food for your systems. They're nourishing and strengthening these systems of the body. And they're all formulations, not a single herb. The ones I use in my practice are customized. There are formulations you can get that are available over the counter that are patent formulas, but they're always in combination, because in Chinese medicine it's never a single herb, it's never a single system you're addressing. This is the brilliance of this Chinese herbal tradition; they understood that to balance the adrenals—at least, to balance the kidney energy, which has a relationship with the liver and the spleen and digestion—all these dynamics must be taken into account to support and balance the whole energetic system. So it's more of a complex science that has been successfully used for thousands of years. I think they're onto something. There are many ways to go, there are many options; this is just my preference because I believe in it. It resonates with me.

But there are formulas out there, adrenal formulas, that are really very good. I would just encourage women to explore this whole world a bit more. If you want to pick something up at the health-food store that's an adrenal support product, there are some good ones, and if you want to investigate the world of Chinese tonics, you can check out a local Chinese practitioner. I did a wonderful interview with a legend in the world of Chinese herbal formulas—his name is Ron Teeguarden—and he introduced the concept of Chinese tonics into the United States in the 1970s. He has a wonderful company called Dragon Herbs (www.dragonherbs .com), and they offer a wonderful service. If you call up, you will get a free consultation with a licensed acupuncturist, and they will listen to what your issues are and recommend formulations based on your symptoms.

NR: If we could line all these things up—if we could clear our adrenal fatigue, rectify any hormonal imbalances, make the endocrine system sing, ensure good digestion, consume the most high-vibration organic substances, sleep well, and have positive relationships—what could the human experience be in terms of longevity?

SS: I believe we could have all our abilities and capacities intact, and just become very wise human beings who are filled with joy and life and vitality, and when our time is up, die happy and healthy. It's a novel concept, isn't it? I spent some time with a Hawaiian elder. She talked about her grandmother, who was a very wise elder. When her grandmother's time to die came, she knew it. She was healthy, but she knew her time was coming, so her family had a big good-bye party for her. Everyone got together and celebrated. Then she went to bed in her best muumuu and never woke up. That to me is a pretty great vision to hold of what we can do, how to have a conscious death and be healthy up to the last minute when it's our time to go. So entertain *that* thought!

NR: That's beautiful. I love the saying, "Look where you're going, because that's where you're headed." When I make decisions today, I like to do them on behalf of my eighty- or ninety-year-old self. Because so much of what we do now is just thinking in the moment, thinking short-term, so putting all these principles of regeneration into practice to serve that stage in our own lives is great.

SS: This is a really important point. The decisions that you make now—whatever now is for you—will determine the quality of your health when you're eighty years old. I have a ninety-year-old mom who has a few little challenges, but she's bright and sharp and really in great health. However, I see how people are in her community. If those people, at eighty and ninety, had realized what their lives would be like, if they could go back in time to where we are, they would make other choices—because we do that have power, and we have to start now. What we do now will determine the quality of our life down the track. Our future selves will be so grateful to our current selves for understanding the responsibility we have to look after our bodies.

The big key for me right now is working with gratitude. Gratitude is such a healing frequency, and the more we can wake up with gratitude for all that we have and go to bed reflecting on all the things we are grateful for, the more we are actually activating the most rejuvenating energy in our bodies. I just encourage people to look around and express that gratitude. It's profound.

To learn more about Dr. Sellman, visit www.whatwomenmustknow.com.

Q&A WITH DR. FRED BISCI

Dr. Fred Bisci, eighty-three, has a PhD in nutritional sciences and has run a practice in New York City for over fifty years. He has worked with more than 35,000 people all over the world with numerous health issues, helping them to heal and regenerate through a clean approach to diet, nutrition, and lifestyle. His protocol draws from biochemical and physiological inter-relationships, and emphasizes "what is left out" versus "what is put in" the human body.

The body is spiritual and vibrationally induced, electrically and chemically empowered, and biologically and genetically carried out.
—Dr. Fred Bisci

NR: If people were to cleanse their bodies and eat a mostly raw, plant-based diet (assuming a clean environment and healthy emotions), what would natural aging look like for us? How long could we live, looking and feeling vibrant?
FB: If we lived in a perfect, pristine environment and everything we ate was clean, we would live far beyond our expectations. The human body is a very specific biological organism, and we are designed to live by natural law. The closer you get to living according to natural law, the better chance you have of living a very long time. But we have only just scratched the surface of living this way. The problem is that we're being bathed in an alien

environment that's highly toxic. We are subject to all kinds of emotional and psychological stresses because of what's going on in the world. Very few people have it all completely together.

If you're eating a vegan, plant-based diet that's either all raw or mostly raw, and you're doing it correctly—a lot of people are not doing this correctly because they don't realize how their body chemistry changes and becomes more sensitive to what's negative over time—your body will evolve and get closer to where it was designed to be. If you consistently try to live a pristine type of diet—not only physically, but also spiritually and emotionally—what happens is, you'll reach a point after a number of years where you develop an elevated consciousness. You become very intuitive, very aware of what's going on.

Everything that we leave out that's not conducive to creating health in the human body to one degree or another corresponds to a reciprocal amount of improvement. Everything that we include that is not meant to be utilized in the human body has a detrimental effect. Processed food is a modern-day curse, and what it does over a period of time is based on your genetic expression—the thoughts you entertain, your spirituality. It will catch different people in different ways. So the key is to understand that the human body is a God-given remedial, biological organism. If you leave out what is offensive to your body, and you cleanse it, there isn't one chronic disease that can't be alleviated very, very quickly. And we know that the body has the ability to overcome some serious diseases. We're very gifted; we just don't realize how gifted we really are.

A lot of people think that nutrition is what heals you. It doesn't. The nutrients that you need enable the body to reach its peak efficiency, but you also have to leave out the substances that are toxifying you, and try to cleanse yourself of past indiscretions. If you do all of that, then miraculous healing can take place. When you cleanse the body and you do it right—and you put it all together with unconditional love, kindness, gratitude—I believe the human life span could be extended far beyond our expectations.

NR: What is your personal health routine and diet?
FB: I've eaten 100 percent raw with no cooked food for over forty-five years. I'm very diligent and disciplined about sticking to my dietary regimen.

NR: Can you tell us what a day in your life looks like, when you're in the center of your power living?
FB: I've had tremendous energy and clarity of mind. Many years ago, I was a big man who weighed 200 pounds. I was very healthy, and I was a weightlifting champion in the Navy, so I didn't get into this because I was sick. I was looking for something. I got into this because I wanted to use my own experience and my own body to find out what was true. I've done short fasts and extended fasts; I've lived on juices. It took me about four years to get comfortable on a raw-food diet. I did lose a lot of weight; everybody was shocked and couldn't understand why I was doing it, since I'd always been a healthy guy. But I always had curiosity. I wanted to be sure that I experienced everything myself and wasn't just going on what somebody said in a book who may never have tried some of this stuff.

Some people say that you can't live on an all-raw diet. I heard one guy who is supposed to be very knowledgeable say this, and his justification was that he tried it and couldn't do it. Well, that's nice, but that doesn't mean other people can't do it, or that it can't be done correctly with dramatic, positive impacts—a longer life that's disease-free (unless something odd happens), clarity of mind, a spiritual awakening. Is a raw diet for everybody? To be honest with you, I don't think so. But if you can do it, and do it correctly, and deal with the social ramifications (some people will look at you like you're an oddball or have an eating disorder), it can be miraculous.

NR: If you were to create a protocol for someone who has already transitioned to a largely raw diet and was asymptomatic, what would that look like for, say, a fifty-year-old woman who wanted to turn back the clock and realign?
FB: I'd want to ensure that she's getting all the nutrients she needs, and that she's also psychologically and spiritually grounded. I would encourage her to use juices, blended salads, and smoothies. She should also be getting an adequate amount of rest, because rest (along with a clean diet) is the ultimate way to help you deal with stress and strains, and to slow down the aging process. She should not be eating late at night—one of the biggest traps for people on raw-food diets—because it creates a fermentation process. Everyone thinks the lower GI tract is the important one, but it's not; the upper GI tract is sixteen to twenty feet, and when you're eating late at night you've got this fermentation that's acid-forming and passing into the blood. Of course there are super-green foods, certain supplements that people can use, but if you're doing this right, you don't really need it.

Then, of course, exercise is a really important catalyst, such as yoga, Pilates, tai chi, qigong, breathing—breath is life-giving. If you're exercising, especially near the ocean or waterfalls, you're getting those negative ions, you feel the difference. The thing is, you don't want to stress yourself with the exercise. You can overdo it, like running marathons—that's not a good idea. It took me time to find that out.

Entertain good thoughts, because bad thoughts will become a reality; try to have an attitude of gratitude in life; try to reach out to help somebody else to make yourself feel better; do those activities that provide true breath and energy. You have to rest and go into anabolism to rebuild and give you strength. Focus on your breath. It restores you, regenerates you. And if you do this right, you'll see changes in your skin. Your skin will tighten up, lines will start to disappear, your hair will get more lustrous. But it doesn't happen overnight; it's an ongoing process.

NR: Being such a maverick in your own family, can you give us some tips on how you were able to stay the course, despite living against the grain, especially around family and friends who think what you're doing is extreme?

FB: I was brought up in an immigrant Italian family. My mother was a fabulous cook, and the Mediterranean diet happens to be a very good diet. I've seen people live to be over a hundred on that type of a diet. I'm very fortunate. My family does not eat the way I do, but they eat a good diet, and they are very supportive of what I'm doing because they see the results on a daily basis. My wife will tell you that she's never seen anyone else who has my energy. Socially, I have no real problems because I socialize with everybody. Someone who's eating the worst type of diet, I have no problem with that—I don't judge people by their diet. If someone has an interest in the way I eat, I will share my experience with them, but I don't want my diet to consume me, to be the only thing I can talk about, because that can alienate people.

NR: Is there anything specific people can do to keep their bones and teeth strong, besides cleansing (taking out the bad stuff and putting in the good stuff)—anything you would say people must do?
FB: Dr. Luigi Fontana did a big study at Washington University Medical School. His subjects were people on a vegan, mostly raw diet. What he found out was that no matter what their age was, their arteries were absolutely pristine, perfectly clear. But he found that *70 percent* of them were suffering from bone-density problems. I think that study has been published. I believe we now have the answers in eating a variety of leafy greens, vegetables, and smoothies, as well as some good form of salt. People with bone-density problems need to be sure they're getting all the minerals and trace minerals (which is not that hard to do) and an adequate amount of protein. Then, of course, they have to exercise to put stress on their weight-bearing bones. If you put that whole package together, your bones will be very strong, and with periodontal care you should have all or most of your teeth for your whole life. It's also very important to chew your food well. Remember, when you put food into your mouth, it sends a message to your brain, indicating which enzymes are best for what's in your stomach.

NR: What are your favorite protein sources for raw vegans?
FB: Nuts, seeds, chia seeds, sesame seeds—there's all kinds of stuff out there. But remember, there's protein in just about everything, especially in green leafy vegetables. One pound of broccoli has 16 grams of protein, so you can blend some broccoli up with other vegetables. You don't really need a lot of supplements. There are raw supplements like hemp protein, spirulina, chlorella—that's perfectly fine to help keep you more heavily muscled, but it's not absolutely necessary. Also chia seeds and sesame seeds. You don't need a lot of nuts and seeds. If you make a smoothie with leafy greens, plenty of berries, maybe some banana, a teaspoon of super greens, a few almonds, a few walnuts, maybe a teaspoon of chia seeds, and coconut water—it's just tremendous. It's a complete meal in itself, providing just about everything you need.

But something that people don't always realize is that if you're on a raw diet, it's extremely important that you keep your internal body temperature up. If you're living in a cold climate and you're feeling cold all the time, you've got to add more calories. You have to keep yourself warm. It's much easier to be a raw-foodist in Costa Rica or Florida, for example, because you're getting plenty of sunshine and radiant heat.

NR: Can you speak a bit about cellulite? Living in the modern environment, knowing that the body is trying to keep toxins away from the vital organs, and fatty tissue seems to be the best receptacle for it, can women who live amidst all the pollution and environmental estrogens fully eradicate cellulite?
FB: It's not easy, and you have to be consistent about cleansing, but yes, absolutely. Remember, oxygen is extremely important for eradicating cellulite. If you get enough oxygen in there and you're being nourished with greens, you can definitely get rid of the cellulite. Yoga, stretching, the right type of massage—this circulates the blood and brings in the enzymes.

NR: Is there anything else you would like to share or add that you think people must know about youth regeneration?

FB: Probiotics are miraculous. If you use them correctly, over a period of time it'll clean out that GI tract, especially the upper GI tract. It'll put billions of the right type of bacteria there that will scavenge and clean everything up—so it won't be fermenting and causing gas and discomfort. Then there are the systemic enzymes, which are unbelievable anti-inflammatories. Most diseases, including aging, commence with inflammation. If you're reducing your inflammation, which systemic enzymes are fabulous for, your aging process will slow down.

To learn more about Dr. Fred Bisci, visit his website, www.anydoubtleave itout.com.

Q&A WITH RICHARD HARVEY

Richard Harvey, seventy years young, has been practicing biological terrain assessment since 1994. He has studied with all the acknowledged masters in the field, including Dr. Robert Young (PhD), Dr. Thomas Rau (MD), and Dr. Marie Blecker (MD). He is certified in biological medicine and homotoxicology, and is a member of the Biological Medicine Network. He works alongside his wife, Mary, sixty-five, a long-term cancer survivor, nutritionist, raw-food instructor, and health coach certified in Ayurvedic medicine. Richard creates personalized health protocols for his clients based on what he sees in their live blood specimens, and Mary inspires them with delicious recipe suggestions to ensure they stick with that protocol. Together they are a dynamic healing team.

> *The name of the game of longevity is to regain control of our biological terrain.*
> *—Richard Harvey*

NR: Would you kindly share your knowledge of hormone replacement and endocrine support as it pertains to rejuvenation?
RH: It is widely understood that hormone replacement therapy (HRT), though effective in producing immediate relief from many symptoms

associated with menopause, is not without problems. Many people have thought that using "natural" bioidentical hormones would not be fraught with the hazards associated with synthetic hormones. The common denominator between synthetic and bioidentical hormones is that they are both exogenously produced and then introduced into the body ecology without reference to the intricate mechanisms for regulating hormonal secretion. This ultimately produces rather intractable regulatory disturbances.

Most hormones work in the body via a negative biofeedback loop. This means that as the level of a specific hormone rises, a signal emanates that ceases the production of that particular hormone. Because of this very sensitive, very accurate hormone-regulating system, when it is circumvented through the introduction of exogenously produced hormones, there are going to be problems.

True, these problems will not occur immediately. In the short term the results may in fact seem to approach the miraculous. However, when you take a hormone, the regulating system will continue to do what it is supposed to do and shut down endogenous production. After a few months go by, it is progressively more difficult to reboot endogenous production, and you are left with an endocrine system which is more dysfunctional than when you began treatment. You are left with a system that should be constantly adjusting to one that is permanently blocked. This does not augur well for health and happiness.

Much has been written about hormone replacement therapy. The present FDA consensus is that HRT can be justified at the onset of menopause in younger women for the relief of symptoms such as hot flashes, vaginal dryness, loss of sexual appetite, and sleeping disorders. It is thought that in cases where there are not mitigating factors, such as a history of diabetes or breast cancer, the risk level is acceptable. The use of hormone replacement for disease prevention, such as heart attack prevention, stroke prevention, osteoporosis, weight gain, and chronic fatigue, is not recommended.

My opinion based on twenty years of clinical observations: Monthly menses is a very efficient way to excrete accumulated acidic toxins, such as environmental chemicals, recreational and pharmaceutical drug residue, inflammatory biological mycotoxins, yeast aflatoxins, and so on. As this natural "chelating" mechanism is phased out, the body activates other mechanisms for keeping pH within functional norms. Pulling calcium from the bones and the resulting progression of osteoporosis is the usual mechanism. Heart attacks and strokes are both due to sclerotic calcification (plaque) buildup in the vascular system. A simple prevention regime for typical postmenopausal calcification "disease" is raising the pH. This will prevent osteoporosis and calcification of the vascular system with its attendant symptoms

Among its many functions, estrogen is a growth hormone. It is for growing babies. Postmenopausal elevated estrogen levels will still tend to promote growth. The question is—of what? We are living in highly carcinogenic times. Our human biology is heavily burdened. Adding estrogen into the mix in order to avert menopausal symptoms does not make sense, especially when there are other options. What these other options are is based on an analysis of a person's individual biology, but could include: hormone-balancing formulas composed of herbs, such as black cohosh and maca for help in the management of hot flashes, night sweats, and related symptoms, along with passion flower, chasteberry, and wild yam. For irritability, anxiety, and insomnia, the adaptogenic herb, ashwagandha, regulates the hypothalamus, pituitary, and the gonadal axis, and thus influences the regulated production of androgen and its mood-stabilizing properties. Homeopathic remedies for symptomatic relief, and isopathic remedies for promoting endogenous regulation, are also part of the mix.

How the life transition called menopause will be experienced is largely a factor of adjusting the biological terrain so that it is as normal as possible in these inclement times. To ease passage through this normal life transition, we must think not just in terms of the symptoms but of the biological context, and making this context as normal as possible. Our neutraceutical protocols are highly individuated. However, for all of our clients, we recommend a daily intake of the following:

- A hydration drink of clean spring water fortified with ConcenTrace minerals, Greens Formula, and Tri-Salts by Ecological Formulas.

- Sulfur-based amino acids, which provide the safest and most effective form of chelation for enabling the excretion of harmful toxins of all kinds—from mercury to mycotoxins to pesticides.

- Antioxidants in the form of vitamins C, D3, and E, which help to protect the cells, tissues, and organs from oxidative stress, and protect vital functions from the destructive effects of toxins of all kinds.

- L-glutamine, which, when combined with NAC (N-acetylcysteine) in the body, results in glutathione, the primary immune modulator.

- A diet of live foods, which is essential for regeneration (cooking food destroys the enzymes necessary for metabolic uptake). The live-food diet should include raw green juices, raw green soups, and wheatgrass juice—the latter being almost 100 percent chlorophyll, and nearly bioidentical to hemoglobin.

- Meditation, because as spiritual and biological beings, our journey back to health and wholeness necessitates the harmonious integration of these complementary aspects of our nature.

Contact Richard Harvey for a live blood analysis and consultation via e-mail at arkgateway@live.com.

Q&A WITH MIMI KIRK

Raw-food chef Mimi Kirk, seventy-five, is a beacon of light for aging naturally. She is the author of *Live Raw* and *Live Raw around the World*. Mother of four and grandmother of seven, Mimi was voted PETA's Sexiest Vegetarian Over 50, at the age of seventy.

> *Feeling like you're in your twenties at seventy-four is quite an amazing thing. I accredit this youthful look and spirit not only to my attitude, but really to my way of eating, which is a raw vegan living-foods lifestyle.*
>
> *—Mimi Kirk*

NR: You have been a vegan for the better part of forty years, and a raw vegan for the last six years. Can you tell us the impact your diet has made on your longevity and beauty today in your seventies? How big of a role do you feel juicing leafy greens has played?

MK: I can truly say that the last six years of being raw vegan took years off my physical appearance and enhanced my health in many ways. Being a vegetarian or vegan can still leave room for eating foods that are not quite healthy. I found eating a raw vegan diet much more in line with clean eating. I think raw food is amazingly delicious. I juice daily, anywhere from sixteen to thirty-two ounces. My basic drink is dark leafy greens (spinach, kale, romaine), celery, cucumber, and apple. I also eat lots of kale and parsley salads. I'm addicted to dark leafy greens.

NR: At an age where most people's organs are weakening and requiring support from medications, kindly describe your vitality and the fortitude of your vital organs and intestine.

MK: I believe age can play a part in the deterioration of the organs if one agrees to let that happen. What I mean is, we can alter that concept if we eat a healthy diet and have a positive outlook about aging. I seem to be healthier than many people in my age group. I know it's not just genes, as research claims genes are only about 5 percent of how well we age or how long we live. My family history includes cancer, high blood pressure, heart problems, Parkinson's, leukemia, and much more. So far at the age of seventy-five, I've managed to prevent these diseases and avoid using medications due to my healthy habits.

NR: What is your take on HRT and bioidentical hormones? Did you take them at any time? If so, what was the result? If not, did you use anything else? What do you recommend on that front?
MK: I'm not a fan of HRT. I've researched and found too many side effects for me to dabble in it. I bypassed all the standard suggestions and went right for monthly acupuncture and Chinese herbs. I was fifty-eight when menopause started, and the most I experienced was hot flashes at times. I also think my mental state was good, as I looked forward to not having to deal with my period anymore. I did not worry about the "change of life," as it's called, and just embraced it as a new and exciting time of life.

NR: Tell us about your relationship with the sun. Do you avoid the sun? Do you embrace the sun during safe hours?
MK: We need sun for vitamin D, but only in the safe part of the day. I always wear sunglasses, which I think are very important, and a hat when I'm out walking around in the hottest part of the day. I use coconut oil on my face and normally will wear long sleeves. Just to add, I do take vitamin D drops, and suggest that everyone should get their blood tested for D and B. If the results are good, it's not necessary to take anything, but if you are on the line or a little low, I recommend a supplement. Even if you eat the perfect diet, your body might not absorb these vitamins, so supplementing is important.

NR: What are your favorite cosmetic items? What do you look for in "youth-regenerating" skin care?

MK: I suppose I'm pretty simple when it comes to skin care. I wash my face daily with Dr. Woods liquid Black Soap, and slather 100 percent coconut oil on my face and body after my bath. I'll occasionally try natural products when people send them to me, but I seem to go back to my own daily routine.

NR: What have been the most essential practices for maintaining your well-being and beauty into your seventies?
MK: I put diet at the top of my list, but there are other rituals I follow and think are very important to live a long, healthy life. I try to walk daily and keep active. I climb stairs many times a day in my home, and I practice yoga. I'm in a happy, committed relationship, and I'm very close to my four children and seven grandchildren. I look at the positive in life and feel grateful for what I have. I'm passionate about spreading the word to others about eating a healthy diet, which I do through my books *Live Raw: Raw Food Recipes for Good Health and Timeless Beauty,* and my soon-to-be-released book, *Live Raw around the World,* and my YouTube channel, where I demonstrate how to prepare raw food. Having a purpose in life is essential to maintaining a youthful spirit.

NR: What does a day in Mimi Kirk's life look like?
MK: I have a large following on social networks, so I try to answer everyone in the morning and sometimes throughout the day. I like to answer interview questions first thing in the morning, or write articles I've been asked to write early in the day. I prefer walking in the morning and yoga later. Once I'm out of bed (that's where I answer people on my laptop), I bathe, get dressed, and make a green juice. I admit I spend lots of time in my kitchen preparing food and trying out new recipes. It's like a hobby for me, and I love the hum of the dehydrator, as I know something good is going on in there. I love shopping at farmers' markets and our local organic farm stand. I look after my vegetable garden and harvest what is ready to eat. My boyfriend and I just purchased bikes, so we are excited to ride a

few times a week. I spend time writing and preparing for talks and demonstrations that I give. They are all different, depending on the audience I'm presenting to. They take time to prepare. I accept only a couple clients on a monthly basis and work with them one or more times a week. I spend time with my family whenever possible, and relax at night with a movie on our large projector screen. We travel quite a bit, and I will jump on a plane at a moment's notice. Travel is one of my favorite things to do. When one feels healthy with boundless energy, life can be fun at any age.

To learn more about Mimi Kirk, visit: www.youngonrawfood.com and her Facebook page.

Q&A WITH TONYA ZAVASTA

Health and beauty expert Tonya Zavasta has authored more than five books about natural beauty and the raw-food diet, including *Your Right to Be Beautiful* and *Quantum Eating.* Tonya has particular expertise in age-defying beauty solutions, and travels the world lecturing on the benefits of the raw-food lifestyle on health, beauty, and longevity. She frequently appears on national television and is featured in numerous magazines.

> *I believe wholeheartedly in cleansing and have made it an integral part of my raw-foods lifestyle. But it's what you do after the cleanse that will make a real difference in your health.*
>
> *—Tonya Zavasta*

NR: Tonya, what's your take on bioidentical hormone replacement therapy? Have you used it? If so, what was your experience? If not, then have you used any herbal or homeopathic remedies instead? What works best along with a largely natural foods or raw-foods lifestyle? What's been your experience with menopause?

TZ: I have no personal experience with HRT at all, synthetic or bioidentical. Nor do I use herbals or homeopathic remedies. "Pleasant" and "menopause" typically don't go together, but that's how it was for me. My mom hit menopause in her mid-forties. A textbook case: mood swings, hot flashes, night sweats, dryness, irritability—the works. I've been eating raw for sixteen years now. That regimen, plus yoga and other exercise, helped me to be ready for menopause well *before* I experienced it. My periods became progressively lighter during the last ten years and then stopped at age fifty-five. It all happened quite uneventfully. And, I'm delighted to say, with *no* discomfort. As in—*none.* That alone, the myriad of other benefits aside, was worth the effort of going raw. And the best part of it . . . the raw-food lifestyle prevents opposite-sex resemblance that inevitably happens after fifty to almost everyone on cooked food.

NR: What is your personal regimen? How do you ensure that your internal organs stay toned and your blood stays alkaline, while living in our acidic modern world?
TZ: I typically have three meals a day. Breakfast: a coconut water–based smoothie with baby bananas and hemp seeds. Lunch, about eleven: fresh juice and a cup of soaked nuts. Dinner is usually a big bowl of salad around two p.m. And that's it. I don't eat or drink until the next morning. I call this eating regimen Quantum Eating (QE). I vary the game with seasonal produce. But otherwise, these three simple meals remain pretty much the same. Most of what I eat is alkaline. This, along with daily fasting and limited quantities, lets me know my blood pH balance is where it needs to be. As far as organ toning goes, there's always yoga.

NR: Is cleansing a part of your regimen?
TZ: Cleansing is downright fashionable these days. I believe wholeheart-edly in cleansing and have made it an integral part of my raw-foods life-style. But it's what you do *after* the cleanse that will make a real difference in your health. After a detox, please don't retox! Once your cleanse is done, up the ante. Make some changes toward increasing your health and your commitment. Cleansing works when you adopt it as a lifestyle rather than

as a sporadic fix. I used to fast regularly, thirty-six hours every week. Since adopting the Quantum Eating method, however, I no longer find it necessary. Why? Because fasting and cleansing are *inherent* in the QE lifestyle.

NR: I understand the whole raw-foods approach, but what's that "rolling pin" thing in your online store? Can it really regrow hair?
TZ: It's the Rolling Bed of Pins, aka the Skin Rejuvenator. It does indeed stimulate hair growth by producing a small galvanic current when the pins, made of different metals, come in contact with your skin. The rolling action causes blood flow to rush to the hair follicles, stimulating and reawakening dormant hair cells. All you'll feel is a warm tingling. Just five or ten minutes a day will do it. But you've got to be consistent—day after day—or you'll lose that improved circulation.

NR: Tonya, what would you say are the most important things a person must do to ensure the integrity of cells, tissues, and bones through the years?
TZ: Just a few core habits will do most of the work. Let me enumerate: Don't eat at night. In fact, this one works, to a degree, *whatever* diet you're on. Skip dinner, or, even better, have it mid-afternoon, and you'll experience more restful sleep, more efficient cell rejuvenation, and a "lighter," happier overall feeling. Once I made two o'clock my last mealtime of the day, my health—already good—improved markedly. This one practice will reset your biological clock like nothing else.
   Eat raw.
   Chew your food thoroughly, extracting every bit of benefit.
   Practice stretching and do some weight-bearing exercises every day.

NR: What would you most like people to know about lasting beauty?
TZ: At age thirty-seven, seeing my droopy eyelids and puffy face in the mirror, I knew I couldn't ignore my declining health any longer. That's when I went raw to slow the aging process. Taking this one step met and

exceeded my expectations. However, eating raw is just one piece of the puzzle. Eating less is another important piece. Raw food is ideal for this, since it is utilized more fully than animal, processed, or cooked foods. Raw fruits and veggies are nutrient-dense, and over time your body will adjust to the smaller amount of food entering your stomach. While raw foods are my main practice, I found that when I hit forty-five, I needed a vigorous beauty routine. Skin aging accelerates significantly after fifty, and you can't rely on raw foods alone to help you look young.

NR: Could you address tooth degeneration?
TZ: Many dentists believe that heredity is a big factor in predicting one's dental condition, and I happen to agree. My father-in-law died at sixty-nine without a single tooth. My mother-in-law, dying from ovarian cancer at seventy-four, had a full set of reasonably healthy teeth even as the rest of her withered away. During their fifty years together, the two of them ate the same food. If genetics is not on your side, then there's a challenge for you: You'll have to care diligently for your teeth. The good news: The result will be a great benefit to your overall health. My book *The Raw Food Diet and Your Compromised Teeth* was written to help people who are going raw to avoid complications they might experience with compromised teeth. In it, I share certain tooth-care practices that can allow one to live a raw-food lifestyle without a single new cavity, and greatly improve the conditions of the gums, especially around root-canaled teeth.

To learn more about Tonya Zavasta, visit her website, www.beautifulonraw.com.

PART VII

The Recipes

JUICES

Fresh, organic, raw, cold-pressed juices are to our cells what fresh, living water is to plants. In today's world, where soil is so depleted of vital nutrients and life force is so much harder to come by in our food, air, and water, juices are nothing short of a saving grace. In our parents' generation, supplements were considered to be the solution to this dramatic decrease in nutritional density in our food supply. Today, juices are finally getting their long-awaited, highly deserved day in the sun. They do what, in my professional opinion, bottled supplements can only pretend to do—truly deliver epic quantities of nutrients and life force to the body in a way that can be instantly and effortlessly assimilated. Raw vegetable juice is the new diet staple for our generation. Drink up the goodness, and feel the difference!

Natalia's Classic Green Lemonade

1 head romaine lettuce or celery

5 to 6 stalks kale (any type)

1 to 2 apples, or 1 to 2 packets of stevia, or liquid stevia drops as needed for sweetness

1 whole organic lemon, whole or peeled depending on taste preference*

1-inch knob ginger (optional)

MAKES 1 SERVING

*The lemon will cut out the "green" taste that some people struggle with.

The Great Eliminator

1 medium or large beet

1 whole cucumber

1 head romaine lettuce

10 medium carrots

1-inch knob ginger (optional)

MAKES 2 SERVINGS

The Great Rejuvenator

2 large whole cucumbers

1 head romaine

1 handful parsley

½-inch knob ginger

1–2 lemons, whole or peeled

MAKES 2 SERVINGS

Clean Bloody Mary

1 small beet

3 carrots

1 orange bell pepper

1 handful parsley

5 stalks celery

1 large whole cucumber

4 Roma tomatoes

½ lemon, with peel

2 garlic cloves

¾-inch knob ginger

Liquid stevia drops (optional)

MAKES 4 SERVINGS

Good Morning Mojito

1 whole English cucumber

2–3 limes, half peeled

1 handful mint

1 head romaine lettuce

Liquid stevia drops to taste

MAKES 2 SERVINGS

The Refresher

1 large whole cucumber

1 head celery

4 leaves lacinato kale (aka dinosaur kale and Tuscan kale)

1 handful cilantro

1 lemon, half peeled

1 lime, half peeled

1 poblano pepper, seeded

½-inch knob ginger

8 ounces fresh coconut water

MAKES 4 SERVINGS

SMOOTHIES

The following recipes are wonderful mid-morning, lunch, or afternoon meal options. You may also enjoy them as dessert after a simple raw meal. Think of smoothies as sweet alternatives to salads. Greens are always a wonderful addition to fruit, so feel free to experiment!

Crystal-Filled Key Lime Pie

2 handfuls baby spinach

16 ounces fresh, raw coconut milk

Juice of 4 key limes (if available) or 2 regular limes

1 teaspoon lime zest (optional)

15–20 drops vanilla stevia

2 tablespoons shredded dried coconut

Blend all the ingredients in a high-speed blender until smooth. For optimal effect, serve this delicate, multifaceted, flavorful smoothie in a crystal cup, glass, or bowl, topped with shredded coconut. It's fairly thick, so feel free to eat it with a spoon or a straw. **MAKES 1 TO 2 SERVINGS**

Green Piña Colada

1 cup fresh chopped pineapple

1 cup fresh young coconut milk

3 handfuls baby spinach

1 cup ice cubes

Blend all the ingredients in a high-speed blender until smooth and enjoy within 12 hours. **MAKES 1 TO 2 SERVINGS**

Pumpkin Pie in a Bowl

This recipe is a detox staple, enticing to raw food lovers and initiates alike. I'm including it here because it is a tried-and-true favorite!

32 ounces fresh carrot juice

1 cup peeled and cubed raw sweet potato

1–2 packets stevia, or drops of liquid stevia to taste

¼–½ avocado

½ teaspoon pumpkin pie spice

Blend all the ingredients in a high-speed blender until smooth and enjoy within 36 hours. **MAKES 4 SERVINGS**

Chlorophyll-Banana Milk Shake

1–2 cups fresh coconut milk

2–3 frozen bananas

2 tablespoons raw mesquite or maca powder

1 teaspoon pumpkin pie spice

2 handfuls spinach

Blend all the ingredients in a high-speed blender until smooth and enjoy within 12 hours. **MAKES 2 TO 3 SERVINGS**

Berry Young

2 cups fresh or frozen blueberries or strawberries

1 cup alfalfa sprouts

1–2 cups fresh coconut milk (or 1 banana with ½ cup coconut or spring water)

Stevia to taste

Blend all the ingredients in a high-speed blender until smooth and enjoy within 12 hours. **MAKES 2 TO 3 SERVINGS**

Sunshine Joy

1 cup alfalfa sprouts

6 organic dates (optional for extra sweetness, or substitute stevia)

2 cups chopped pineapple

3 leaves kale, de-stemmed

1–2 tablespoons packed fresh mint

Blend all the ingredients in a high-speed blender until smooth, adding a few ice cubes as necessary to prevent the mixture from warming up during blending. This smoothie is best served immediately, but it will keep in the fridge for up to 2 days.

MAKES 2 TO 3 SERVINGS

Carob-Spinach-Banana Shake

Enjoy this super-indulgent yet super-light dessert following an avocado salad, or just on its own for lunch or a mid-afternoon energy booster!

1 box organic baby spinach (about 4 ounces)

2 boxes organic alfalfa sprouts

2–3 ripe frozen bananas (or unfrozen, but frozen for an "ice cream" texture)

4 heaping tablespoons pure carob powder

1½ cups raw young coconut water or pure water

Stevia to taste

1½ cups ice cubes

Dried shredded coconut (optional)

Apple pie spice (optional)

Blend all the ingredients except the shredded coconut and apple pie spice in a high-speed blender until smooth, adding a few ice cubes as necessary to prevent the mixture from warming up during blending. This smoothie is best served immediately, but it will keep in the fridge for up to 2 days. If desired, top with shredded coconut and/or apple pie spice before serving. **MAKES 3–4 SERVINGS**

RAW SAVORY SOUPS

Raw Roma and Basil Soup

2 Roma tomatoes, diced

10 kalamata olives, diced

2 beefsteak tomatoes, quartered

1 bunch basil

1 avocado, pitted and peeled

Stevia to taste

1 teaspoon agave nectar (optional)

Sea salt to taste

Combine the diced Roma tomatoes and olives in a bowl and set aside. Blend all the other ingredients in a high-speed blender until smooth. Add the diced tomatoes and olives into the blended base and enjoy within 12 hours. **MAKES 2 SERVINGS**

Curry Corn Soup

4 cups fresh corn cut off the cob (about 4 to 5 large ears)

¼ cup diced red bell pepper

1 jalapeño pepper, finely diced

1 cup organic almond milk (Pacific brand is recommended)

1 cup vegetable broth

1 avocado, pitted and peeled

3 teaspoons curry powder

2 teaspoons finely minced Spanish onion

Sea salt and pepper to taste

5 drops or 1 packet stevia

Set aside ¼ cup of the corn, the red bell pepper, and the jalapeño pepper. Blend all the other ingredients in a high-speed blender until smooth. Add the reserved corn and the peppers and enjoy within 12 hours. **MAKES 4 SERVINGS**

Avocado Soup and Salad

½ small cucumber, peeled

Juice of 2 lemons

2 handfuls of greens (e.g., sprouts, spinach, or other tender baby greens of choice)

1 handful parsley

1 avocado, pitted and peeled

Sea salt to taste

Optional toppings:

Dulse (red seaweed) flakes

Raw agave

Nama Shoyu soy sauce

Sweet paprika

Blend all the ingredients in a high-speed blender until smooth and enjoy within 12 hours. Add the optional toppings before serving if desired. MAKES 1 SERVING

Ginger Ivory Splendor Soup

Flesh and water of 2 raw young coconuts

1 cup cubed raw butternut or acorn squash

10 drops or 2 packets stevia

1 knob peeled ginger root, diced

1 teaspoon sea salt

2 tablespoons vanilla extract

Blend all of the ingredients in a high-speed blender until smooth and enjoy within 12 hours. MAKES 4 SERVINGS

SALADS AND SIMPLE RAW CREATIONS

Each of the following Raw Regeneration Bowls is a totally satisfying, life force–rich meal in a bowl. And, if I do say so myself, each one is an intuitive masterpiece of maximum flavor and vitality!

Raw Regeneration Bowl #1: The Amazing Marinara Cell-Cleanse

For the salad base:

1 medium zucchini, peeled into ribbons with a vegetable peeler

1 medium summer squash, peeled into ribbons with a vegetable peeler

1 large carrot, peeled into ribbons with a vegetable peeler

4 ounces organic baby romaine lettuce

For the marinara:

5 Roma or vine-ripened tomatoes

5 unsulfured sun-dried tomatoes, soaked in 1 cup of purified water for 10 minutes

1 tablespoon fresh oregano

¼ cup packed fresh basil

1 tablespoon fresh rosemary

1 heaping tablespoon fresh ginger, diced

2 cloves fresh garlic

2 tablespoons cold-pressed olive oil

1 teaspoon Nama Shoyu or Tamari soy sauce

1 teaspoon Himalayan or Celtic sea salt (or to taste)

Stevia to taste

Combine all the salad base ingredients in a large bowl. Place all the marinara ingredients in a high-speed blender and blend until smooth. Pour the blended marinara mixture over the vegetables in the bowl. Toss, serve, and dig in! **SERVES 2**

WOODEN BOWLS AND CHOPSTICKS

Personally, I prefer to serve my meals in wooden bowls with wooden utensils, ideally wooden chopsticks. I find that eating with metal forks, spoons, and knives—all the stabbing, shoveling, and cutting—creates an aggressive disconnect between me and the food that I am asking to replenish and heal me. This is why I make sure to eat with a peaceful heart and mind, with a feeling of love and gratitude. (Even the best alkaline foods will turn acidic if consumed in a negative spirit.) I will resort to normal cutlery when necessary while eating out, but there is nothing like wooden bowls and chopsticks to present your meal in the most gentle, natural, and healing light.

Raw Regeneration Bowl #2: Wild Herb, Sprout, and Dandelion Power with Quick Tahini Dressing

For the salad base:

1 cup organic sunflower sprouts

½ cup packed dandelion greens

4 ounces baby romaine or baby mixed lettuces

2 tablespoons fresh parsley

2 tablespoons fresh basil

For the dressing:

1 cup raw tahini

¼ cup fresh lemon juice

1 clove garlic

1 tablespoon ginger, diced

1–2 teaspoons Nama Shoyu or Tamari soy sauce

Stevia to taste

Place all the salad base ingredients in a bowl. Blend all dressing ingredients in a high-speed blender and pour on top of the salad. Toss and enjoy—creamy and scrumptious!

SERVES 1–2

TIP FOR BLENDING

Since the blending process heats up the precious ingredients of dressings and raw soups, adding a few ice cubes to the blender before blending helps to preserve the mixture's freshness and integrity. This is especially important for ingredients that are better served cool, such as that beautiful raw tahini!

Raw Regeneration Bowl #3: Carrot-Ginger Live Forever

4 ounces baby romaine lettuce

1 cup grape tomatoes, halved

1 cup sunflower sprouts (substitute alfalfa sprouts if necessary)

1 ripe Hass avocado, sliced

½ bulb fennel (optional)

10 ounces fresh carrot juice

3 tablespoons fresh lemon juice

2 cloves garlic

2 heaping tablespoons fresh ginger

Stevia to taste

Himalayan or Celtic sea salt to taste

Combine the lettuce, tomatoes, sprouts, avocado, and fennel (if using) in a bowl. In a high-speed blender, blend the carrot juice, lemon juice, garlic, and ginger until smooth. Pour the mixture over the vegetables. Sprinkle on some stevia and/or sea salt as desired, toss, and serve. **SERVES 1–2**

Natalia's Favorite Raw Salad

    4 generous handfuls baby romaine lettuce and/or baby spinach

    ½ cup cherry tomatoes, halved

    3 ounces raw goat cheddar, grated (Alta Dena is a good brand)

    ¼ cup fresh lemon juice

    Stevia to taste

    1 tablespoon diced fresh garlic

    Fresh herbs (optional)

Toss all the ingredients together in a large bowl and serve. You can season the salad with fresh herbs such as basil, oregano, rosemary, or chives, or grated beet, for a more gourmet flavor, but it is simply delicious on its own. **MAKES 2 TO 4 SERVINGS**

Tender Baby Salad

Jerusalem artichoke is what is known as a prebiotic, meaning it provides optimal food for activating healthy bacteria in the gut. This delicious salad is soft and tender, and an aid to digestion.

    2 cups lamb's lettuce (aka mache or corn salad)

    2 cups baby lettuce

    ½ cup alfalfa or broccoli sprouts

    ½ cup grape tomatoes, halved

    ½ cup cucumber, finely sliced

    1 Jerusalem artichoke, finely sliced

    ¼ cup fresh dill, chopped

    ¼ cup fresh lemon juice

    Stevia to taste

    1 teaspoon diced fresh garlic

Toss all the ingredients in a large bowl and enjoy! **MAKES 4 SERVINGS**

Creamy Avo-Ranch Salad

Salad:

¼ cup alfalfa sprouts

1 red or orange bell pepper, julienned

¼ medium cucumber, thinly sliced

2 cups baby mixed greens

Dressing:

½ avocado

1 beefsteak tomato

1 tablespoon finely chopped parsley

1 tablespoon finely chopped cilantro

½ cup apple cider vinegar

2 cloves garlic, diced

1 tablespoon Dijon mustard

5 drops or 1 packet stevia

Toss all the salad vegetables in a large bowl. Blend all the dressing ingredients in a high-speed blender until creamy. Pour the dressing over the salad, lightly toss, and serve. MAKES 2 SERVINGS

Harvest Salad

½ red onion, diced

1 large carrot, thinly sliced

1 cucumber, peeled and diced

½ cup sliced Jerusalem artichokes (matchstick pieces)

¼ cup packed fresh mint

4 cups spring lettuces

4 tablespoons balsamic vinegar

¼ cup cold-pressed olive oil

½ cup whole walnuts

10 drops liquid stevia

1 teaspoon nutmeg

1 teaspoon cinnamon

½ cup thinly sliced dried figs

Toss all the vegetables and lettuce in a large bowl with the vinegar and olive oil, withholding one tablespoon of the oil. In a separate bowl, drizzle the remaining oil over the walnuts, then sprinkle with the stevia, nutmeg, and cinnamon, and mix until the nuts are coated. Toss the walnuts into the salad with the dried figs and serve. **MAKES 4 SERVINGS**

Mama Mia Pizza Salad

6–8 unsulfured sun-dried tomatoes, soaked and chopped

½ pound fresh baby greens

3 ounces shredded raw cheddar-style goat cheese

2 tablespoons raw sheep pecorino

¼ cup chopped basil

1 tablespoon chopped oregano

2 tablespoons dried parsley

2 tablespoons apple cider vinegar

10 drops or 2 packets stevia

2 cloves garlic, thinly sliced

Sea salt and pepper to taste

Mix all of the ingredients in a large bowl and serve. **MAKES 2 SERVINGS**

Classic Avocado Salad

½ pound mesclun greens

1 ripe avocado, diced

1 cup quartered grape tomatoes

Juice of 1–2 lemons

1 tablespoon diced fresh garlic

Sea salt and fresh pepper to taste

Stevia to taste

2 tablespoon diced sweet onion (optional)

Toss all of the ingredients together in a bowl. The mix of the creamy avocado with lemon and stevia makes for the simplest gourmet meal. To make it divine, toss the salad until the avocado creates a creamy dressing. MAKES 2 TO 3 SERVINGS

Mexican Salad

3 heads romaine lettuce, finely chopped

2 cups finely chopped yellow bell peppers

4 tomatoes, chopped

½ cup raw corn off the cob

½ red onion, diced

¼ cup chopped cilantro

1 diced jalapeño pepper

Juice of 2 limes

2 tablespoons cold-pressed olive oil

10 drops or 2 packets stevia

Toss all the ingredients together in a large bowl and enjoy. MAKES 2 TO 4 SERVINGS

Tahini Delight

Salad:

½ pound romaine or baby spinach, chopped

2 bell peppers, thinly sliced

2 carrots, cut into matchsticks

Dressing:

½ cup raw tahini

1 tablespoon Nama Shoyu or Tamari soy sauce

½ teaspoon sea salt

1–2 garlic cloves

½-inch knob ginger

Juice of 2 limes

1 tablespoon coconut water

Stevia to taste

Combine the romaine, peppers, and carrots in a large bowl and set aside. Blend all of the dressing ingredients in a high-speed blender until smooth, then toss into the salad until evenly coated. MAKES 2 TO 4 SERVINGS

Simple Pasta Puttanesca

5 vine-ripened tomatoes

⅓ cup packed fresh basil

⅓ red bell pepper

¼ cup fresh oregano (optional)

1 tablespoon minced fresh ginger

1½ cloves garlic

½ small red onion, diced

¼ cup pitted kalamata olives

Juice of ½ lemon

½ cup sun-dried tomatoes

Celtic sea salt and freshly ground pepper to taste

1 large zucchini or spaghetti squash, spiralized or julienned into fine strips

Blend all the ingredients, except the zucchini or squash, in a high-speed blender until creamy. Pour the tomato sauce over the zucchini or squash and serve. MAKES 4 SERVINGS

Green Log in the Sun

1 stalk celery

1 teaspoon raw almond butter

½ teaspoon raw honey

Cinnamon powder to taste

Sunflower sprouts

Spread the almond butter on the celery stalk, drizzle on the honey, add a sprinkle of cinnamon, and garnish with sprouts. Enjoy! MAKES 1 SERVING

Raw Goat Cheese Sandwich

2 tablespoons marinara sauce

6 romaine lettuce leaves

6 thin slices raw cheddar-style goat cheese

Spread a small amount of marinara sauce on each lettuce leaf, and top each one with a slice of cheese. Roll into a tube and munch! MAKES 2 SERVINGS

Simple Raw Guacamole

This basic recipe is a great dip for a plate of chopped raw vegetables (crudités).

2 ripe avocados, peeled, pitted, and mashed

1 tomato, diced

1 red onion, diced

1 jalapeño pepper, seeded and diced

1 bunch cilantro, chopped

1 red pepper, seeded and chopped (optional)

Juice from 1 lemon or lime

1 pinch sea salt

Combine all the ingredients in a bowl and mix well with a fork. Serve fresh. MAKES 2 SERVINGS

Tip: If storing overnight, squeeze a little extra lemon juice on top of the guacamole to keep it from browning.

FROM THE HEARTH

Mediterranean Beet Salad

Cooked veggies make a satisfying addition to a raw salad. Beets are not only delicious but also help to activate the bowels if you're feeling stuck. Enjoy this hearty salad at night, and feel liberated the next morning!

    7 small to medium beets, washed and trimmed
    2 small boxes baby spinach
    6 ounces crumbled goat or sheep feta
    1 cucumber, julienned
    1 handful dill, chopped
    2 garlic cloves, minced
    Juice of 2 lemons

1. Preheat the oven to 400°F.
2. Wrap the beets in wax-free paper sandwich bags or foil, and bake them for 1 hour.
3. Roll the beets on the countertop while still in their bags, or shake them in a large paper bag to remove the skins.
4. Quarter the beets and toss them with the remaining ingredients in a large bowl and serve.

MAKES 2 TO 3 SERVINGS

Note: You may serve the beets warm, or cool them in the fridge for 1 hour.

Sweet Potato Toast

    2 sweet potatoes, cut lengthwise into ¼-inch-wide strips
    Sea salt
    Herbes de Provence

Preheat the oven to 400°F. Bake the sweet potatoes on a lightly greased baking pan for 20 minutes, flipping them halfway through. Serve them as a side to any avocado-based salad. **MAKES 1 TO 2 SERVINGS**

Sweet Butternut Heaven

 3 cups cubed butternut squash

 1 to 2 packets stevia (as desired for sweetness)

 2 teaspoons pumpkin pie spice

 2 teaspoons organic butter

 Sea salt to taste

Preheat the oven to 350°F. Combine all of the ingredients together in a mixing bowl and evenly distribute onto parchment paper on a baking tray. Bake uncovered for 35 minutes, or until the squash cubes are soft and brown on the edges. Serve hot. **MAKES 2 SERVINGS**

Spicy Curry

 ½ cup vegetable broth

 ½ cup coconut milk

 2 cups cauliflower florets

 ½ cup sliced shiitake mushrooms

 ½ cup julienned carrots

 ½ cup snow peas

 ½ onion, diced

 1 tablespoon diced garlic

 1 tablespoon diced fresh ginger

 1 jalapeño pepper, diced

 4 tablespoons curry powder

Heat the vegetable broth in a wok or a skillet. Add all the remaining ingredients, cover, and cook over low heat for 5 to 10 minutes, or until the vegetables are soft. Pour the curry mixture into large bowls and serve. **MAKES 2 TO 4 SERVINGS**

Garlic "Bread" Goat Melts

1 globe eggplant, sliced into ½-inch-thick rounds

Garlic powder to taste

Sea salt to taste

2 ounces goat mozzarella or raw goat cheddar, shredded

Preheat the oven to 400°F. Place the eggplant rounds on a lightly greased baking pan, season with garlic powder and sea salt, and bake for 8 minutes on each side. Top the eggplant with the goat cheese and bake for another 2 minutes, until the cheese is melted. Enjoy! **MAKES 2 SERVINGS**

Quickest Spaghetti

This recipe is a basic detox staple that is great for beginners. It is easy, satisfying, and delicious.

2 large zucchinis, sliced into pasta-like strips with a mandolin or a spiralizer

½ cup organic pasta sauce*

½ cup raw goat cheese, grated (optional)

In a small saucepan, heat the pasta sauce well and pour over the zucchini. Toss and top with the goat cheese if desired. **MAKES 2 SERVINGS**

* Note: The Seeds of Change and Paesana brands are the best-tasting and healthiest bottled sauces I have found (the Muir Glen is very pure but is not as tasty), and they are easy to find in the local health-food store. Other organic high-quality pasta sauces are acceptable, too, but look for little to no sugars (never refined sugars) or oil (only olive oil) listed as one of the last ingredients.

Color Melt

 2 unpeeled zucchini, grated

 2 unpeeled summer squash, grated

 2 large carrots, grated

 1 head broccoli, cut into florets

 1 cup shiitake mushrooms, whole or sliced

 1 cup organic marinara sauce

 4 ounces raw cheddar-style goat cheese, grated

1. Preheat the oven to 250°F.

2. On the stovetop, steam the zucchini, squash, carrots, and broccoli in a steamer and heat the pasta sauce in a saucepan.

3. When the vegetables are soft, arrange them in a baking dish, topped with the mushrooms and the heated marinara sauce. Sprinkle with cheese and place the whole dish in the oven with the door ajar for 3 minutes, or until the cheese has melted.

4. Serve hot and enjoy!

MAKES 2 SERVINGS

Eggplant Pizzas

 4 eggplant rounds, thinly sliced

 Sea salt and pepper to taste

 ½ cup organic tomato-basil pasta sauce

 4 ounces raw cheddar-style goat cheese, grated

 ¼ cup chopped fresh basil or oregano (optional)

Toast the eggplant rounds on a baking tray in the broiler until lightly brown on both sides. Meanwhile, heat the pasta sauce. Remove the eggplant from the broiler and top with the sauce, cheese, and chopped herbs. Return to the broiler until golden, and serve hot. **MAKES 2 SERVINGS**

LES POTAGES

Grain-Free Asian Kombu Noodle Soup

This is a great cold-weather soup. It really heats you up inside!

  3 cups organic vegetable broth

  1 cup julienned carrots

  1 cup thinly sliced lotus root (optional)

  1 cup sliced shiitake mushrooms

  1 tablespoon minced fresh ginger

  1 tablespoon minced fresh garlic

  1 tablespoon soy sauce (Nama Shoyu if possible)

  2 packets soft Kombu seaweed noodles, rinsed*

  ½ cup snow pea shoots**

1. In a large soup pot, combine all of the ingredients except the Kombu noodles and the snow pea shoots.

2. Bring the ingredients to a boil. Reduce the heat, cover, and let simmer for about 10 minutes until vegetables are very soft and have flavored the broth.

3. Ladle the soup mixture evenly on top of the Kombu noodles in a large serving bowl, and garnish with the snow pea shoots. Serve hot.

MAKES 4 SERVINGS

* Sea Tangle kelp noodles are soft and pasta-like, packed in water and ready to use. If you cannot find Sea Tangle kelp noodles easily at your health-food or gourmet grocery, you may order them online at kelpnoodles.com or amazon.com.

** Snow pea shoots are available in most gourmet stores and farmers' markets, but if you cannot find them, they may be omitted.

Vegetable Soup Perfection

As with all homemade soups, the longer the vegetables soak in the broth, the more flavorful the soup will become. This soup can sit in the refrigerator for up to four days. For a thicker soup, you may blend half the mixture, then add it back to the batch. Feel free to add any other vegetables that you love.

8 large carrots, chopped

5 stalks celery, chopped

1 leek, chopped

1 head broccoli, chopped into florets

1 zucchini, chopped

1 cup chopped baby bella mushrooms

1 cup chopped okra

½ medium onion, chopped

Equal parts water and organic vegetable broth to cover vegetables (about 6 cups)

½ serrano chili, diced (optional)

Spike seasoning to taste

Curry powder to taste

Celtic sea salt to taste

Place all the ingredients into a large pot and bring the mixture to a boil. Reduce the heat, cover, and simmer for 5 to 10 minutes, or until the carrots are semisoft. Serve hot with sprouted-grain toast with organic butter and/or raw honey. **MAKES 4 SERVINGS**

Creamy Parsnip Soup

15 parsnips, chopped

32 ounces organic vegetable broth

1 small Spanish onion, chopped

2 to 3 cloves garlic, chopped

1 tablespoon dried sage

1 tablespoon dried parsley

1 tablespoon sea salt

Place all the ingredients in a pot, bring to a boil, cover, and reduce to low heat. Cook until the parsnips are soft. Let the mixture cool and then puree in a high-speed blender. Serve hot, or freeze for an easy reheatable meal during a busy week. **MAKES 4 SERVINGS**

Comforting Carrot and Sweet Potato Soup

This soup is so easy—minimal chopping required!

> 2 sweet potatoes
>
> 2 cups baby carrots
>
> 1 cup water
>
> 2 cups organic vegetable broth
>
> ½ teaspoon Celtic sea salt
>
> 1 packet stevia
>
> ¼ teaspoon cumin
>
> ½ teaspoon coriander powder
>
> ¼ teaspoon minced ginger
>
> ¼ teaspoon minced garlic

Bake the sweet potatoes in their skins for 30 to 45 minutes at 450°F until soft, and boil the carrots until soft. De-skin the potatoes. In a blender, mix all the ingredients until smooth. Pour the mixture into a large saucepan and heat on the stovetop. Serve hot.

MAKES 4 SERVINGS

SEAFOOD

Simple Spiked Snapper

   2 half-pound red snapper fillets

   2 tablespoons fresh-squeezed lemon juice

   1 tablespoon organic butter

   1 clove garlic, diced

   Spike seasoning to taste

Preheat oven to 450°F. Place the fish in a baking dish, add the lemon juice, dab the fillets with butter, add the garlic, and sprinkle on some Spike seasoning to taste. Cover with a lid or aluminum foil and bake for approximately 25 minutes, or until the fish begins to flake. Serve hot. **MAKES 2 SERVINGS**

Detox Maple-Glazed Salmon

This dish is ideal for entertaining. It's quick and easy to prepare, and quite possibly the juiciest, most flavorful dish your friends will ever taste!

   1 cup Nama Shoyu or Tamari soy sauce

   1 clove garlic

   1 tablespoon minced fresh ginger

   1 tablespoon toasted sesame oil

   1 tablespoon pure maple syrup (or liquid Stevia if preferred)

   4 fresh salmon fillets, well rinsed

1. Mix the soy sauce, garlic, ginger, sesame oil, and stevia in a blender until the mixture reaches a smooth marinade consistency.

2. Spread the soy sauce mixture over the fish evenly in a baking dish. Cover and marinate the fish in the refrigerator for 1 to 24 hours.

3. Preheat the oven to 450°F. Bake the fish for about 18 minutes, or until it flakes easily with a fork.

MAKES 4 SERVINGS

Scallop Consommé

6 large wild scallops

1 onion, chopped

2 cloves garlic, chopped

1 large carrot, diced

2 Roma tomatoes, diced

¼ cup chopped fresh parsley

¼ cup sliced scallions

5 cups water

1 teaspoon white wine

1 teaspoon lemon juice

Celtic sea salt and freshly ground black pepper

Place all the ingredients in a soup pot and bring to a boil, then reduce to a simmer over low heat for 35 minutes. Enjoy hot. **MAKES 2 SERVINGS**

EGGS

Western Omelet

    1 teaspoon butter

    ¼ cup chopped bell pepper

    ¼ cup chopped onions

    ¼ cup chopped mushrooms

    ¼ cup chopped tomatoes

    4 organic free-range eggs

    ½ cup grated raw cheddar-style goat cheese

    Fresh baby greens (optional)

1. Melt the butter in a skillet over medium heat. Add the vegetables and cook until slightly brown. Transfer into a bowl.

2. Whisk the eggs together and pour into the same hot skillet used to sauté the vegetables. Cook for 2 minutes, and add the vegetables back onto the eggs.

3. Top with the cheese and cook until the eggs are no longer runny and the cheese is melted. Fold the omelet over and remove from heat. Enjoy with lots of fresh baby greens.

MAKES 1 SERVING

Ana's Favorite Frittata

    6 organic free-range eggs

    2 tablespoons water

    2 tablespoons grated raw sheep pecorino

    ½ tablespoon olive oil

    2 Roma tomatoes, sliced

    ¼ cup grated raw cheddar-style goat cheese

    1 small bunch fresh basil leaves

1. Beat the eggs well with the water and the pecorino.

2. Grease a cast-iron skillet or a pie dish with olive oil and fan out the tomato slices to cover the bottom.

3. Cover the tomatoes with the goat cheese and basil leaves. Pour the egg mixture into the pan to cover the tomatoes, cheese, and basil.

4. Bake for 20 minutes or until golden brown and a knife pulls out of the center cleanly.

5. Slice the frittata into quarters and serve warm or chilled.

MAKES 4 SERVINGS

Sweet Choco-Crepes

¼ cup soft goat cheese (aka chèvre)

10 drops liquid stevia

1 teaspoon cocoa powder

1 teaspoon butter

4 organic eggs

Sea salt

1 pinch cinnamon

1. In a small bowl, mix the goat cheese, stevia, and cocoa powder into a sweet chocolate paste.

2. Melt the butter in a skillet over medium heat. Whisk the eggs together and pour into the hot skillet. Cook for 2 minutes, and add the goat cheese and cocoa paste, evenly distributed over half of the omelet. Use a crepe-maker if you have one, but this is really delicious even in more of an omelet form.

3. Lightly salt and cook until the eggs are no longer runny and the cheese is melted. Fold the omelet over and remove from heat. Sprinkle with cinnamon and sea salt and serve hot.

MAKES 2 TO 4 SERVINGS

DESSERTS

For the raw ice creams, all you need is a good blender. Place all the ingredients plus 1 cup of the ice in a K-Tec blender or other high-power blender. Begin blending on #4, or at the highest speed. Gradually add the remaining ice as long as the mixture is flowing and blending well (you may have to run it two or three times during this process). You need not use all the ice—just enough to make the mixture thick. You may also wish to use a little coconut water to facilitate blending.

Raw Chocolate Ice Cream

    3 bananas

    3 tablespoons pure cocoa powder (I recommend Green & Black and Shiloh Farms)

    2 tablespoons organic raw, unsalted tahini or almond butter

    6 organic dates, pitted (or stevia to taste for the yeast-conscious)

    3–4 cups ice cubes (about 14 cubes)

    MAKES 4 SERVINGS

Raw Vanilla Ice Cream

This is a divine rendition of regular vanilla ice cream.

    Meat of 3 young coconuts

    1 tablespoon pure vanilla beans

    ½ cup pure maple syrup (or 1 tablespoon + stevia to taste)

    4 cups ice cubes (about 14 cubes)

    MAKES 2 TO 4 SERVINGS

Raw Chocolate Raspberry Ice Cream

This is a deeply satisfying raw and dairy-free treat that is just as creamy and delicious as a pint from your local grocery store. This recipe is a variation of my Raw Strawberry Ice Cream, which is the most popular of all my ice creams. (To make the strawberry version, simply swap the frozen raspberries for frozen strawberries, omit the cocoa powder, and use strawberry extract.)

   Meat of 2 raw young coconuts

   2 ten-ounce bags frozen organic raspberries (I like the Cascadian Farm brand)

   Liquid stevia to taste (approximately 10 to 20 drops)

   3 tablespoons pure cocoa powder (I like Green & Black or Shiloh Farms)

   6 organic dates, pitted (optional)

   1 teaspoon organic raspberry extract

   4 cups ice cubes (about 14 cubes)

   MAKES 4 SERVINGS

Raw Strawberry Sorbet

   2 bags frozen strawberries

   1–2 cups young coconut milk

   Vanilla stevia to taste

   MAKES 4 SERVINGS

Cheat Tiramisu

   ¾ cup Laloo's Vanilla Snowflake goat's milk ice cream

   ½ tablespoon pure organic cocoa powder

   ½ tablespoon finely ground espresso beans

If you are feeling extra indulgent, after the ice cream has thawed for 5 to 10 minutes, you can crumble a couple of whole-wheat graham crackers on top and mix them in by hand. **MAKES 1 SERVING**

Raw Chocolate Pudding

This is a simple, classic dessert for the detox lifestyle.

> Meat of 2 coconuts (or ½ an avocado)
>
> 4 dates or stevia to taste
>
> 4 tablespoons pure cocoa powder

Blend all the ingredients in a food processor until smooth. Delicious! MAKES 2 SERVINGS

Detox Minty Hot Chocolate

This is a delicious, satisfying, sweet way to end the day, or transition away from coffee. If the mint and chocolate combination does not please your palate, omit the peppermint extract for a more classic taste, or try another extract in its place. Vanilla, orange, and raspberry are all delicious options.

> 2 cups boiling water
>
> 2 tablespoons 100 percent cocoa powder
>
> 2 tablespoons carob powder (optional)
>
> 1 pinch sea salt
>
> 10 drops peppermint extract
>
> Stevia to taste

Combine all the ingredients in your favorite mug, stir, and enjoy! MAKES 1 SERVING

CONCLUSION

Take a moment to think about how the Taoist Masters and Shaolin monks live, and how their fabled ancient ancestors lived. They maintain a higher order of life, based on ritual, simplicity, and a closeness with nature. They breathe the most vital mountain air, drink water from living springs that originate in the magnetic depths of the Earth. They eat wild and simple foods. They are not pulled this way and that by the strings of commercial culture. They don't give their energy and life force to countless modern distractions, or collude with a lifestyle that wears them down. They do not congest their lives with convoluted rules, credit card bills, traffic, acidic substances, and an overload of possessions. They do not race like rats up corporate ladders or consider stress a normal state of being. Nor do they obsess about weight loss and anti-aging fads. And yet, they are famed for their longevity and youthfulness.

Most of us, on the other hand, have taken for granted that the modern paradigm is the only way to live. I hope that this book has shown you that there is another way. A way to regenerate your cells and your spirit continually as you circle the sun. A way to reveal your most vibrant, authentic self. A way to shine at any age. Syncing up with nature's powerful rhythms brings fulfillment on the deepest levels. It means loving more, laughing more, being more inspired, more innovative, more relaxed—and, yes, it means becoming more beautiful and youthful. Choose the unobstructed path of regeneration, and you will move through the world with enviable freedom.

We know a great deal about the degenerating effects of our modern lifestyle. We have all experienced its terrifying dissonance—physically, emotionally, and spiritually. Like the proverbial frog in a pot of boiling water, so many of us have spent far too long being cooked. But it turns out that what we thought were the inevitable indignities of aging are actually the result of modern living. If we can jump out of the pot and find a more natural habitat, a way of life that is more attuned to who we are and what we are made of, then we can save ourselves from premature ruin.

Remember, the philosophy of timeless beauty is quite simple: *To experience the grace and vitality of youth, we must flow with nature, not against it.*

What is less simple is integrating this wisdom into the busy lives we lead. Of course, many of us are tempted by the glossy promises of modern medicine, the shortcuts to beauty and youthfulness. Many of us live in cities and towns where cars, computers, and wireless technology rule the day. I am not about to trade in my life for the secluded existence of a Buddhist monk, however much I may admire and crave that path at times. Nor do I expect this of you. However, I am confident that as you incorporate more and more of the principles and practical applications of timeless beauty into your everyday life, you will start to experience profound changes. Then, you can take them further, continually shedding old cells and blockages to allow for new growth.

To all the doomsayers out there, I say that nature is still alive and well. It is within and all around us. It's just a matter of seeing it, honoring it, tapping back into it. Let's reach for our highest good, remaking ourselves as we would remake the world we live in. External beauty and youthfulness are but the expressions of inner health and vitality. Wisdom and connection. Love and understanding. I wish all of this for you, dear reader. May you be forever young, beautiful, and radiant on your continual journey around the sun!

ACKNOWLEDGMENTS

In a world with very few examples of humans becoming more beautiful and light-filled with age, I have been extremely fortunate to witness, learn from, and be inspired by several such rare individuals. My biggest influence has been my own mother, who has set the gold standard for how to live the golden years for me. In addition, there was my dear friend, Helen Kulnik, who passed away recently at the ripe age of ninety-five—but not without first showing me how sparky, clear, and energetic one could be at that stage of life.

Pioneers of longevity Mimi Kirk, Tonya Zavasta, Almine, Fred Bisci, and Richard and Mary Harvey have each paved their own vibrant futures, of which I've taken grateful and precise note. Because of them, I have a real sense of direction for my future. Their dedication to truth has shown me how to move forward through life on my own terms, without compromise. I also thank them sincerely for sharing their knowledge in this book.

I would like to express my enormous thanks to Dr. Eric Braverman and Dr. Jon Turk, who so generously took time away from their busy Manhattan practices to allow me to interview them. Both are remarkable doctors with an enviable passion for their work—I admire and appreciate them greatly!

Younger, but not least, there are the two women who made this book possible. My editor, Anna Bliss, who has been beside me for the better part of the last decade, and my dear friend, Ana Ladd-Griffin. It was Anna Bliss who insisted that I could indeed complete this book, despite my concerns about writing it while managing DetoxTheWorld and a growing family. Her extraordinary ability to transform my often wildly unwieldy concepts into silky sentences amazes me time after time. Were it not for her confidence in me and her determination to bring this information forward, this book would not have been possible. Ana Ladd-Griffin has also been at my side for more years than I can keep track of as my staunchest ally. Ana spent endless hours researching and perfecting several sections of this book. I can't imagine how *Forever Beautiful* would ever have seen the light of day without her focused efforts.

Forrest Beaumont, my dear friend and genius photographer, took the cover photo for this book. He is a prince among men, and his rarefied eye has resulted in so many beautiful photographs over the years, including this one.

I want to thank my husband, Lawrence, who has made sure every door has remained open to my dreams; that the mundane tasks of everyday life never stand in my way of achieving them. Lawrence is my knight on a white horse if ever a girl had one!

Finally, I want to thank our children, Thandi, Tommy, and Electra, who fill me with the joy of the universe and reinforce for me every day what is truly precious and life-generating.

FOREVER BEAUTIFUL SHOPPING GUIDE

This shopping guide includes products mentioned throughout the book that I recommend to my clients for regenerative purposes. The following products are by no means mandatory for regeneration beauty and youthfulness; they are merely offered as recommended sources of support and enhancement, for anyone with the desire and the means to seek them out. Although some of the products listed below are admittedly quite expensive, it is because they are of the highest quality and will offer a good value in the long run. Most of the products listed in this guide can also be found in the DetoxShopping section of detoxtheworld.com.

ALTERNATIVE MEDICINE

BECK PROTOCOL

SOTA products are specifically designed for following the Beck Protocol, a natural health, bioelectric protocol designed to help the body heal itself. SOTA carries a Silver Pulser, Magnetic Pulser, Water Ozonator, Bio Tuner, and LightWorks for micropulsing, colloidal silver, pulsed magnetic fields, ozonated water, and light for "health and harmonic frequencies." They come with clear directions, and video tutorials are available. The SOTA products are easy, personal-use products of the highest quality (endorsed by Bob Beck himself). They can be ordered directly from www.sota.com.

CHINESE HERBS

Dragon Herbs are the wonderful Chinese herbs Dr. Sherrill Sellman refers to in her interview, which I've personally used to nourish my female essences after three pregnancies. They are available online through www.dragonherbs .com. Dragon Herbs is based in Santa Monica, California, where they have a storefront. Trained acupuncturists are on call to help you select the best herbal blends to support your unique needs.

PROBIOTICS

Dr. Ohhira Probiotics should be taken as directed, alone and on an empty stomach (ideally in the morning before your green juice, or else in the late afternoon before dinner). For more information, or to order them directly, visit drohhiraprobiotics.com, or order from www.detoxtheworld.com or www.amazon.com.

Ascended Health probiotic drops are another great way to cultivate healthy intestinal flora for optimal digestion. They are available directly from www.ascendedhealth.com, as well as from www.detoxtheworld.com.

PROGESTERONE CREAM

Emerita Pro-Gest is the fragrance-free, paraben-free progesterone cream I used when I needed to rebalance my estrogen dominance after prolonged nursing. It is available online at www.emerita.com, as well as most health-food stores.

APPLIANCES

BLENDERS

BlendTec and Vitamix are brands of industrial-strength blenders that make any blended recipe fast and easy. They are easy to clean, and have long-lasting blades and motors. Both brands are sold on amazon.com, or can be purchased directly from the manufacturers at www.blendtec.com and www.vitamix.com.

JUICERS

Breville Juice Fountain juicers are our longtime favorite for ease of use and cleaning, longevity, and for Breville's customer care and generous replacement and repair policies. They are sold on amazon.com, directly from www .brevilleusa.com, or from www.detoxtheworld.com. They are also available at Williams-Sonoma and Bed Bath & Beyond.

BEAUTY / PERSONAL CARE PRODUCTS
DEODORANT
Nourish Organic Deodorant and Lavanila Laboratories' The Healthy Deodorant are the only aluminum-free organic deodorant products I've found that actually work. While I prefer soap and water, these are great for the occasions that require odor protection. Nourish offers a variety of scents as well as unscented sticks at www.nourishorganic.com. Lavanila products can be found at Sephora or at www.lavanila.com.

MAKEUP
The Urban Decay Naked Palette eye-shadow collection boasts an array of wonderful neutral colors and is 100 percent vegan and cruelty-free (including the brush). It can be found at Sephora, or ordered directly from www.urbandecay.com.

Youngblood Mineral Cosmetics Pressed Individual Eyeshadows are individual eye shadows made from a talc-free formula, with rice starch and mica for smoothness and long wear. They have no perfumes or chemical dyes, and are all-natural and vegan. They can be ordered directly from www.ybskin.com, where you can also find a store locator.

Chantecaille offers a range of cosmetic products that are not tested on animals, have no animal derivatives or synthetic colors and fragrances, and do not contain any sulfate detergents, phthalates, or petrochemicals. The Radiance Gel Bronzer is a favorite of mine. Chantecaille products can be found at Barneys, Neiman Marcus, Bergdorf Goodman, and other department stores, or ordered directly from www.chantecaille.com.

Jane Iredale PureMoist LipColour lipstick is based on micronized minerals and made without fillers, bonders, talc, mineral oil, chemical dyes, or preservatives. It can be ordered from shopjaneiredale.com or found at Nordstrom and at salons and spas all over the world, including SoHo Sanctuary in New York City.

Hourglass is a cruelty-free company that is paraben-free, vegan, and gluten-free wherever possible. The Hourglass Aura Sheer Lip Stain is a staple of mine, which I use on the cheeks instead of the lips as a light, long-lasting blush. Find the right shade for your skin color, and you'll have a double-duty product that can enhance both lips and cheeks. Hourglass products can be found at Sephora, or ordered directly from www.hourglasscosmetics.com.

Caudalie makes a range of skin-care and makeup products that are free of bad chemicals and made with ingredients such as apricot butter, grape-seed oil, and lemon water. Their tinted moisturizers and lip and eye colors are wonderful, ethical products that support some incredible environmental projects and are never tested on animals. Caudalie can be found at Sephora or ordered directly from us.caudalie.com.

INIKA Certified Organic Liquid Mineral Foundation boasts organic antioxidants, vitamins, and minerals and is 100 percent vegan. It provides great long-lasting coverage, unlike many other natural foundations I've tried. The products from this new Australian company will soon be widely available in the United States. INIKA foundation and other products can be found at www.inikacosmetics.com.

Sisley Paris is a French company that uses natural plant extracts to make great products. Sisley Paris Transmat Botanical Makeup with Cucumber Extract is a botanical moisturizing foundation that gets rave reviews from women of all ages. It is infused with soothing cucumber extract for red or irritated skin, and offers really natural coverage. It can be found at Neiman Marcus, Bergdorf Goodman, and Saks. For more retailers, visit their store locator at www.sisley-cosmetics.com.

Nvey Organic Mascara is the only organic mascara I've tried that matches the performance of many mainstream mascaras. It uses organic jojoba oil, beeswax, and carnauba wax, and also smells lovely! It can be ordered directly from www.nveymakeup.com.

NAIL POLISH

Priti NYC nail polish is 100 percent vegan, organic, biodegradable, and never tested on animals. Manufactured in New York City, it offers the same long-lasting finish as chemical polishes. It can be found at ABC Carpet & Home, as well as many other retailers worldwide. You can order it directly from www.pritinyc.com, where you can also find a store locator to see where it is distributed in your area.

DENTAL CARE

Living Libations has a selection of essential oils and a line of tooth-care products that can be ordered from www.livinglibations.com. They are free of fluoride and harsh, abrasive agents.

Tonya Zavasta's Beautiful On Raw dental-care products, such as Bentonite Oral Balm, are available from her website (www.beautifulonraw.com).

Desert Essence Natural Tea Tree Oil & Neem Toothpaste can be found at most health-food stores, including Whole Foods, or ordered directly from www.desertessence.com.

Tate's Natural Miracle Toothpaste is naturally fluoride-free and suffused with peppermint, spearmint, sage, rhatany root, geranium, clove stem, birch-tree extract, eucalyptus leaf oil, papaya extract, and menthol. Tate's is the toothpaste your whole family will love. I also find it whitens the teeth as advertised! I get mine at my local health-food store, but it can also be found online at www.ourtatefamily.com.

DIET AND NUTRITION

DARK CHOCOLATE

Endangered Species offers a variety of dark chocolate bars that can be found at most health-food stores in the United States, including Whole Foods, or ordered directly from chocolatebar.com.

The Rose Bar, our own 70 percent handcrafted Belgian dark chocolate, is produced in small batches and shipped from a secluded exotic beach village in South Africa. It can only be ordered from www.detoxtheworld.com.

Rapunzel German chocolate is 100 percent organic and much creamier at 70 percent cacao than other products. It can be found at most health-food stores internationally, or ordered from www.internaturalfoods.com in the United States. Visit www.rapunzel.de/uk to find distributors on every continent.

Fine & Raw Chocolate is a 100 percent raw chocolate. This delicious treat can be found at many health-food stores, or ordered directly from www.fineandraw.com.

FAVORITE RAW AND DETOX-FRIENDLY TREATS

Didi's pies are a delicious treat for those living a mostly raw detox lifestyle. They can be found in limited selection at some health-food stores, or ordered directly from www.bakingforhealth.com.

Coco-Roons can be find at some health-food stores, some Whole Foods stores, or ordered directly from http://cocoroons.cloudwaysapps.com.

Anke's muffins from The Juicy Naam are delicious, and can be ordered from www.thejuicynaam.com.

GOAT'S MILK ICE CREAMS

Laloo's offers slow-churned 100 percent goat's milk ice cream with a social and environmental certification. It's also certified as a Women's Business Enterprise in partnership with Astra Women's Business Alliance, as a woman-owned business effectively managing a successful company. Find a store near you via www.laloos.com/locator, or order the product online at www.icecreamsource.com.

Victory Garden NYC has fresh goat's milk soft-serve ice cream made with "local ingredients and lots of love." Their buttery ice cream is inspired by the tradition of Anatolian *dondurma:* Turkish goat's milk ice cream made with the root of the wild orchid. Visit www.victorygardennyc.com.

RAW ICE CREAMS

Organic Oasis offers a delicious raw ice cream that can be found at limited health-food stores or ordered directly from www.myorganicoasis.com.

Raw IceCream Company offers nut-based raw ice creams that can be found at Whole Foods or ordered directly from www.rawicecreamcompany.com.

Organic Nectars Cashewtopia ice cream can be found at many health-food stores throughout the United States, or ordered directly from www.organicnectars.com.

RAW SOY SAUCE

Ohsawa Nama Shoyu soy sauce is different than other soy sauce (including Tamari) because it is a raw fermented product. It can be used with any Asian-inspired dish, and has a delicious salty flavor. Nama Shoyu soy sauce can be found at most health-food stores, including Whole Foods, or ordered from www.shoporganic.com.

STEVIA

NuNaturals stevia is simply the best-tasting brand of stevia available. Clear stevia comes in a plastic squeeze bottle that is perfect for the kitchen and for purse or travel. NuNaturals also makes vanilla, cocoa, and other flavored stevias. It is available throughout the United States at GNC, and can be ordered from www.detoxtheworld.com, or directly from www.nunaturals.com.

Pure Green Stevia Powder by Nature Products is for those purists out there who want to use absolutely unadulterated stevia. All you'll find here is finely ground green stevia leaf. I recommend this form of stevia to my clients who, for various health reasons, or out of mere preference, abstain from any alcohols or additives of any kind. It smells and tastes like green tea. I enjoy the earthy purity of it very much. Nature Products Pure Green Stevia can be purchased on Amazon.com.

WILD FISH

Wholey (www.wholey.com) offers a large variety of wild-caught fresh fish fillets and uses gel packs made specifically for seafood to ensure that your fish is perfect upon arrival.

Lummi Island Wild (www.lummiislandwild.com) offers buying clubs all over the United States. They fish in complete harmony with the environment, using an ancient fishing method creating no air, water, or noise disturbance. They are the only solar-powered salmon fishery, and have the ability to return non-target species unharmed to the sea.

EXERCISE

INVERSION BOARDS

Ironman and Health Mark inversion boards get the highest reviews for durability across the board (no pun intended!). Both can be found at www.amazon.com, or directly from the manufacturers at www.healthmarkinc.net/store, and www.ironman-inversion-tables.com.

REBOUNDERS

Bellicon is the top brand on the market for bungee-cord rebounders. I find the Bellicon rebounder to be bouncier and gentler on the skeletal system than the spring-based models. It allows you to jump higher and get a better workout. JumpSport offers a more affordable bungee-cord model. You may purchase one online at www.bellicon-usa.com or www.jumpsport.com.

Founded by Al Carter, ReboundAIR is one of the oldest rebounder manufacturers who make a wonderful spring-based rebounder and truly practice what they preach. They have several models available for easy home storage, and provide video guides for maximizing use. They are available directly from www.reboundair.com, or at a discounted rate from www.detoxtheworld.com.

HAIR CARE

Tela Beauty Organics makes a line of hair treatment and styling products, including shampoos and conditioners targeting many different types of hair (oily, dry, damaged, etc.). The Volume Shampoo and Conditioner and Beach Hair Style Texturizing Paste are wonderful! These products can be ordered from www.telanyc.com, or can be found at Nordstrom and other department stores.

Carol's Daughter Rosemary Mint Clarifying Sulfite-Free Shampoo is a great natural clarifying product for hair that has been in the pool, over-processed, or weighed down with too many products. Most other clarifying shampoos contain very harsh ingredients, so this is a nice alternative. It can be found at Sephora and many drugstores, including Rite Aid, or ordered directly from www.carolsdaughter.com, where you can also find many great products for coarse and curly or African-American hair.

MEDITATIONS AND LECTURES

For your convenience, we have consolidated all the meditations we recommend on www.detoxtheworld.com's DetoxShopping site under Audios

& Meditations. You may also visit the recommended teachers' sites independently:

For Guy Finley's lectures, visit www.guyfinley.org.

For Anita Briggs's meditations and courses, visit www.innermasterytools .net.

For Almine's lectures, courses, and meditations, visit www.spiritual journeys.com.

For audios and classes by Lee Harris, visit www.leeharrisenergy.com; by Story Waters, visit limitlessness.com; by Peggy Phoenix Dubro, visit www .emfbalancingtechnique.com.

SKIN CARE

ARGAN OIL
Pure argan oil from ArganUSA can be ordered from the DetoxShopping section of www.detoxtheworld.com, or from www.zamourispices.com.

BODY BRUSHING
Yerba was founded by a health-conscious group in Northern California who were dedicated to learning the benefits of internal cleansing. The Yerba Prima natural bristle body brush can be found at health-food stores throughout the United States, including Whole Foods, and ordered from www.amazon.com and directly from www.yerba.com.

CEDAR OIL
The Ananda Apothecary carries pure cedarwood essential oils steam-distilled from the wood of wild cedar grown in both Morocco and Nepal, as well as Texan and Virginian cedarwood oils. You may find them at www.ananda apothecary.com.

The Ringing Cedars of Russia carries pure Siberian cedar oil, as referenced in the Anastasia books. You can order from them directly, or find an international and US list of distributors on their website (www.ringing cedarsofrussia.org).

COCONUT OIL

Look for raw, cold-pressed filtered coconut oil from any health-food store, including Whole Foods. Barlean's, Nutiva, and Garden of Life oils can be ordered directly from www.barleans.com, www.nutiva.com, and www.garden oflife.com, respectively.

CUPPING

Venus Body Sculpting Cups are available at www.beautifulonraw.com. Bellabaci cups for the face are available at www.bellabaci.co.za. The NCN Pro Skin Care Vaculifter, a skin- and body-cupping massager, can be ordered from www.ncnskincare.com.

DERMAL ROLLING

Tonya Zavasta describes her Beautiful On Raw Amazing Skin Rejuvenator as a "rolling bed of pins." It causes a minor trauma to the skin, which forces it to regenerate, reportedly increasing blood flow and oxygen while stimulating collagen production, helping the skin of the body tighten and thicken while healing scar tissue and dissolving cellulite. It can also stimulate hair growth when used on the scalp.

MRS Derma Micro Needle MicroNeedle Roller is a smaller, finer model used for the more-delicate skin of the face and neck. It has fine, diamond-shaped needles (less painful than round needles) and uses titanium instead of surgical steel for less possible bending. It also has more needles per roller than other models, making it more effective. Roller the entire face, avoiding the eye and mouth area, vertically, horizontally, and then diagonally for maximum effect. It can be ordered directly from www.skinbeautysolutions.com.

ESSENTIAL OILS

Nothing can harmonize me faster than taking in a deep breath of pure essential oils. I love the Young Living Everyday Oils Essential Oil Collection, a kit that comes with nine of the most popular oils. I put a few drops in my palm, rub my palms together, and just breathe in the fragrances. A little peppermint on the belly can aid a stomachache almost immediately, and a few drops of lavender in the bath or on your chest can facilitate a deep sleep. This essential oils kit is available online at www.youngliving.com.

FAR-INFRARED SAUNAS

High Tech Health high-quality saunas come in several wood options, are easy to assemble at home, and use only nontoxic food-grade adhesive. They are available from the DetoxShopping section of www.detoxtheworld.com, which will guide you directly to the sauna page of www.hightechhealth.com.

MUD AND CLAY

Aztec Secret Indian Healing Clay and Pure French Green Clay Powder are the purest detoxifying face and body clays we have found. They can both be found on www.amazon.com, or ordered directly from www.theportugal onlineshop.com and www.aztec-secret.com.

POST-SUN SKIN-RECOVERY TREATMENTS

JASON Soothing Aloe Vera Organic Oil, Aubrey Organics Aloe Vera Gel, and Made from Earth Pure Aloe Vera Skin Treatment are 100 percent pure, organic post-sun skin-recovery products. Both JASON and Aubrey Organics products can be found at many health-food stores, including Whole Foods, or ordered directly from www.aubrey-organics.com and www.jason-personalcare.com. Made from Earth products are less widely available, but can be ordered directly from www.madefromearth.com.

Skin Trip is a great post-sun skin-recovery moisturizer made with a blend of aloe vera, coconut oil, and lanolin. This light, sweet-scented product can be found at most health-food stores, including Whole Foods, or ordered directly from www.mountainocean.com.

ROSE OIL

RoseGlow Serum by Living Libations can be ordered from www.living libations.com.

SCRUBBING GLOVES

Earth Therapeutics gloves are excellent for exfoliation and stimulating blood flow on the surface of the skin. Earth Therapeutics uses organic natural ingredients whenever possible, and their products can be purchased from many health and beauty retailers, including www.amazon.com, Bed Bath & Beyond, Kohl's, and directly from www.earththerapeutics.net.

SERUMS AND BALMS

Beautiful On Raw Nourishing Night Cream and Facial Cream with Sea Buckthorn Oil are thoughtfully blended, ultra-pure creams that will make you look and feel beautiful instantly. They can be found at Tonya Zavasta's website, www.beautifulonraw.com, along with her recommended five-step skin-care protocol.

Decléor Aromessence Essential Balm and Aromessence Angélique Nourishing Serum can be found at Amazon.com, Nordstrom, or ordered directly from www.decleor.com (even internationally).

Fresh's Crème Ancienne and Elixir Ancien are two favorite new finds that I absolutely love. Both can be ordered directly from www.fresh.com or www.amazon.com.

The Body Deli offers a selection of botanical body lotions and body soufflés that can be ordered directly from thebodydeli.com.

Dr. Hauschka's Regenerating Serum and Regenerating Day Cream are light but effective moisturizing and skin-clarifying products that can be found at most health-food stores, including Whole Foods, or ordered directly from store.drhauschka.com.

For sun damage recovery, vitamin C–based products are extremely helpful. Avalon Organics Vitamin C Renewal Vitality Serum can be found at most health-food stores, including Whole Foods, or ordered directly from www.avalonorganics.com, where the company also provides a guide to locating a local distributor of their products.

SOAPS

South of France French Milled Vegetable Soaps are made of all-natural vegetable ingredients, including organic shea butter and natural moisturizing glycerin, and essential oils and fragrance. They are sodium lauryl/laureth sulfate-, EDTA-, paraben-, and phthalate-free. They can be found at health-food stores throughout the United States, including Whole Foods, and ordered from www.amazon.com, or directly from www.goodhealthnatural products.com.

Trader Joe's French milled soaps are a wonderful budget-friendly alternative, with all-natural ingredients and using the traditional French-milled process.

SUNSCREENS
In my opinion, zinc oxide is the purest form of sunscreen (in fact, it's my sunscreen of choice for my children). While it sounds like a chemical, zinc oxide is found in nature as the mineral zincite. Badger Zinc Oxide Sunscreen Cream is manufactured using 100 percent clean recycled zinc left over from other processes, and purified via distillation into pharmaceutical-grade zinc oxide. Unlike some zinc oxide sunscreens, this brand does not leave the skin looking chalky. Badger products can be found online at www.badgerbalm .com, as well as in most health-food stores.

Juice Beauty offers a variety of organic sunscreen products, including a water-safe SPF 30 Sport Moisturizer and lip sunscreens that can be ordered directly from www.juicebeauty.com.

Josie Maran Argan Daily Moisturizer is a light argan oil–based cream with an SPF of 40. It can be found at Sephora, or ordered directly from www.josiemarancosmetics.com.

VITAMIN E OIL
NOW Solutions Vitamin E oil is widely available at health-food stores, pharmacies, Whole Foods, and online. Trader Joe's also makes its own brand of pure concentrated Vitamin E oil.

YEAST AND FUNGAL TREATMENTS
CANDIGONE
Renew Life CandiGONE is a powerful candida-fighting supplement, and one of the few that are recommended as a complement to the detox lifestyle.

It can be found at many health-food stores, including Whole Foods. It can also be purchased directly from www.renewlife.com, or ordered from www.detoxtheworld.com and www.amazon.com.

GRAPEFRUIT SEED EXTRACT

NutriBiotic GSE, or any other pure grapefruit seed oil, can be taken with green juice for a light citrus flavor, or alone in water for a fungal treatment (following the recommended dosage). It can be found in most health-food stores, or ordered directly from www.nutribiotic.com.

OREGANO OIL

Pure oregano oil is a safe, widely used, and powerful antifungal product. Use two to three drops under the tongue daily on an empty stomach or as directed by the manufacturer. Oregano oil can be found at most health-food stores, GNC, The Vitamin Shoppe, and ordered from amazon.com, or you can purchase it directly from www.oreganoworld.com.

INDEX

ABOUT THE AUTHOR

Natalia Rose is a clinical nutritionist, the founder of DetoxTheWorld.com, and the author of *The Raw Food Detox Diet, Raw Food Life Force Energy, Detox 4 Women,* and *The Fresh Energy Cookbook.* In her private practice, Rose works with some of the world's most body-conscious men and women, including models, actors, and media personalities. She lives in New York City with her husband and three children.

Also by Natalia Rose

The Raw Food Detox Diet
Raw Food Life Force Energy
Detox 4 Women
The Fresh Energy Cookbook